D0777929

beating
the **years**

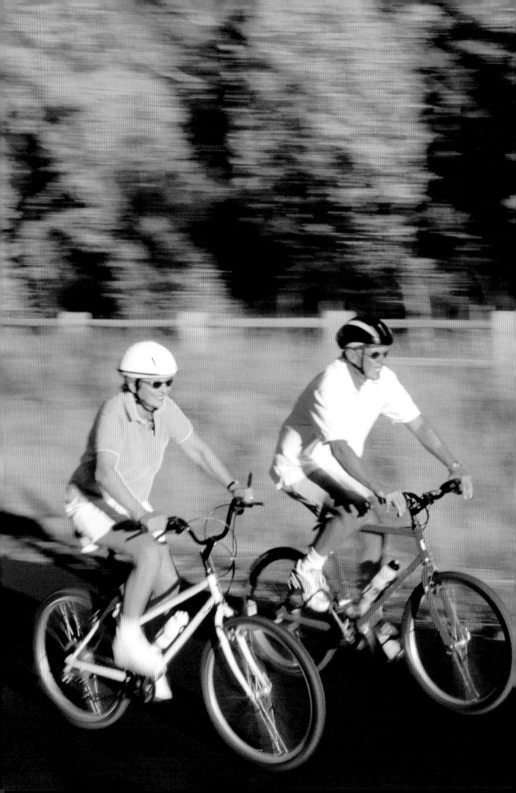

options for health

beating
the years

helen barnett

Dr. Len Saputo, Editor
Richard I. Gracer, M.D., Consultant

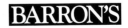

First edition for the United States and Canada published in 2002 by
Barron's Educational Series, Inc.

Text copyright © 2002 Octopus Publishing Group Ltd
Design copyright © 2002 Octopus Publishing Group Ltd

Author's and publisher's note: Before following any advice or exercises contained in this book,
it is strongly recommended that you consult your doctor if you have any symptoms of illness, any
diagnosed health problem, or are taking any conventional medicines for any condition. Do not
stop any conventional treatment without consulting your doctor, and always check with your doctor
or pharmacist before taking a herbal remedy if you are taking any type of conventional medicine
(prescription, or over-the-counter), as they may interact. The publishers and author cannot accept
responsibility for any injuries or damage incurred as a result of following the advice given in
this book.

Additional titles in the *Options for Health* series:
Beating Sports Injuries
Boosting Your Digestive Health

All inquiries should be addressed to:
Barron's Educational Series, Inc.
250 Wireless Boulevard
Hauppauge, NY 11788
http://www.barronseduc.com

Library of Congress Catalog Card Number 2001096143

International Standard Book Number 0-7641-1900-1

Picture Credits
Front cover Stone/Peter Correz; 2 Photodisc; 10 Corbis Stockmarket/Jose Luis Pelaez Inc.; 15 Corbis
Stockmarket/Michael Keller; 17 Photodisc; 23 Photodisc; 31 ImageState/Stock Image; 37 Photodisc; 39
Science Photo Library; 43 Photodisc; 47 Corbis/Jacques M. Chenet; 48 Photodisc; 50
Stone/Michaelangelo Gratton; 56 Octopus Publishing Group Ltd./Hamlyn/Jeremey Hopley; 61
Photodisc; 62 Photodisc; 67 Corbis/RF; 70 Corbis/Claudia Kunin; 73 Octopus Publishing Group
Ltd./Hamlyn/Nick Walker; 76 Photodisc; 79 Corbis/Steve Chenn; 84 Stone/Chris Craymer; 87
Photodisc; 93 Photodisc; 97 ImageState/Stock Image; 101 Corbis/L. Clarke; 105 Photodisc; 110
Science Photo Library/Francoise Sauze; 113 Science Photo Library/Andrew McClenaghan; 116
Photodisc; 121 Octopus Publishing Group Ltd./Hamlyn/Colin Bowling; 125 Corbis/Layne Kennedy; 129
Photodisc; 133 Science Photo Library/BSIP Collet

Printed and bound by Toppan Printing Company, China
9 8 7 6 5 4 3 2 1

contents

Foreword...6

Introduction...8

Part 1:
Understanding Aging

Why do we age?   12

Identifying your aims   14

When to see a doctor   16

Kicking bad habits   20

Heart and circulatory diseases   22

Diabetes   28

Back pain   30

Arthritic conditions   34

Osteoporosis   36

Menopause   38

Prostate problems   40

Sexual problems   42

Memory loss   44

Eye and ear problems   46

Part 2:
Options for Health

Taking care of yourself   52

Nutrition and healthy eating   54

Vitamins and minerals   58

Keeping in shape   64

Simple exercises to do at home   68

Sports   72

Posture   74

Stress   78

Relaxation techniques   82

Sleep and insomnia   88

Skin care   92

Healthy hair   96

Therapies   98

Acupuncture   100

Massage   104

Osteopathy and chiropractic   108

Reflexology   112

Yoga   114

Aromatherapy   120

Herbal medicine   122

Homeopathy   126

Naturopathy and hydrotherapy   130

Conventional medicine   134

Plastic surgery   138

Useful organizations   140

Glossary   141

Index   143

foreword

Throughout history, a healthy lifestyle has been the primary cornerstone for good health—this remains true today. However, we have entered a new and exciting era of incredible technological advances, which can take us beyond mere lifestyle to enjoy a whole new level of vitality. We have the unique opportunity to blend what we have always known with the miracles of new age scientific breakthroughs.

Being young has different meanings for different people. For some, chronological age, the appearance of their skin, hair, and physique, their energy level, the way they dress, their state of health, and behavior, are all factors used to define youth. For others, aging gracefully is a quality respected as a rite of passage associated with great wisdom. It is possible to enjoy both of these perspectives.

Helen Barnett separates fact from fiction as she takes us on an exploration that clarifies what aging is and how we can live our lives with health and vitality. She begins with the fundamentals—what you can do on your own that is simple common sense in order to avoid aging prematurely. The epidemic of chronic degenerative diseases that we now face is taking a horrendous toll on our health by limiting both the quality and length of our lives. There is a lot that you can do to prevent or reverse these illnesses, and *Beating the Years* outlines these solutions in an easy-to-understand style.

This book provides information on both mainstream medicine and a wide variety of complementary and alternative disciplines. Options for treatment can be blended from the style that you choose, which meets your particular individual needs, and at your own pace. The pros and cons of each discipline are presented fairly, and the therapies described are accompanied with simple explanations about how they work. Attention is given to the science behind each healthcare style without dismissing the lengthy history of ancient wisdom that has survived hundreds and, in some instances, even thousands of years.

We were designed with tremendous reserve function in every organ system. However, these reserves are not infinite and once lost, our ability to function may become compromised, leading to disability and even premature death. Poor diet, obesity, lack of exercise, high levels of stress, inadequate sleep, toxic exposures, and lack of meaningful purpose in life all predispose to conditions such as heart attacks, strokes, diabetes, hypertension, depression, arthritis, osteoporosis, and even cancer.

Special attention is given to our habits and addictions such as smoking, alcohol, caffeine, and the drugs that are so commonly used in our lives. In our fast-paced society we look for quick remedies for everything from colds and cancer to the stresses in our lives that lead to anxiety and depression. We are learning that we can and should take responsibility for our health in all domains—physically, emotionally, and spiritually—whenever possible. After all, who is going to be more interested in our well being than us? And, who else can change the style in which we live our lives?

All too often, many of us do not take the time to evaluate and modify these simple fundamentals that have served humanity so well for millennia. Doctors and patients alike have awakened to the reality that when we assume responsibility for our own healthcare we will be healthier. Recent surveys document that over 90 percent of physicians agree that diet, exercise, and stress reduction are major factors in maintaining optimal health.

Working in partnership with your healthcare practitioners is very important. There is much to gain from the years of experience they have spent in training and in clinical practice. However, only you can take responsibility for changing your lifestyle. The buck stops with you, not with your practitioners. The most powerful strategy for beating the years is to merge the wisdom of your healthcare practitioner with your willingness to take responsibility for your own lifestyle.

Dr. Len Saputo, Editor

introduction

Myths and legends abound concerning elixirs for eternal
youth and magic formulas for immortality but, unfortunately,
none of them are true. For the time being, there is no quick
fix to staying young. However, there is lots you can do to
keep yourself fit and healthy, young at heart, and looking
more youthful than you are. This book gives you an insight
into the many ways you can change your diet and lifestyle
to improve your well being into old age. It also gives advice
on what conventional medicine and complementary
therapies can do to help you "beat the years."

While many people stay fit and healthy well into their later years, some develop
chronic diseases associated with aging, such as heart problems, diabetes, arthritis,
or osteoporosis. A chronic health condition can age people much faster than
"normal." However, if you do have a long-term health problem, don't give up hope.
There are many things you can try that, while they might not cure you, can help to
relieve your symptoms, increase your life expectancy, and improve your mobility and
well-being. This section looks at the most common conditions associated with
getting older and briefly outlines some of the therapies, both conventional and
complementary, that might help you. However, always remember that if you have
any persistent, recurrent, or unexplained health problem or your symptoms worsen,
you should consult your doctor.

All the conventional medicines mentioned in this book can have side effects,
and you should find out what these are, and report any you experience to your
doctor or pharmacist. You should also find out about any known interactions
between complementary and conventional medicines before you devise a regime.

As a general rule, this book takes Western medicine and science as the "gold
standard," since this is what most readers will be familiar with. In the West, it is this
conventional medicine that has undergone the most extensive testing and research.

Many alternative therapies are not susceptible to this type of analysis, and where research has been carried out it is often not yet sufficient to be "scientifically" conclusive about the therapy's efficacy. The text of this book will, where appropriate, indicate the level of research undertaken into different therapies. Where it states that there is little scientific evidence to support a treatment, it may simply be because the research has not yet been carried out; similarly there may be little scientific evidence dismissing a specific therapy. However, many complementary medicines and therapies have been practiced for thousands of years, and have the weight of tradition and anecdotal evidence to support them, even though they may not have passed a particular test in a Western laboratory.

Life expectancy

Taoists believe that 100 years is the normal life span for a human being, with 150 years being considered as a long life. At the end of the nineteenth century, the average life expectancy was only about 50 years. In industrialized societies today, however, the average life span is about 75 years for a man and 80 years for a woman, but scientists are predicting that humans could soon live as long as 120 years. This book may not help you to achieve such longevity but it can show you how to help yourself to have a long and healthy life.

How the tabs work

Following the sections on specific conditions and health problems in Part One, Understanding Aging, are a series of colored tabs. These guide you to the most appropriate therapies that are most likely to be useful for treating a particular condition or health problem, and relate to the color coded sections in Part Two, Options for Health. In this section you will find more detailed information on the suggested therapies.

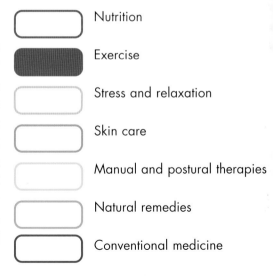

Nutrition

Exercise

Stress and relaxation

Skin care

Manual and postural therapies

Natural remedies

Conventional medicine

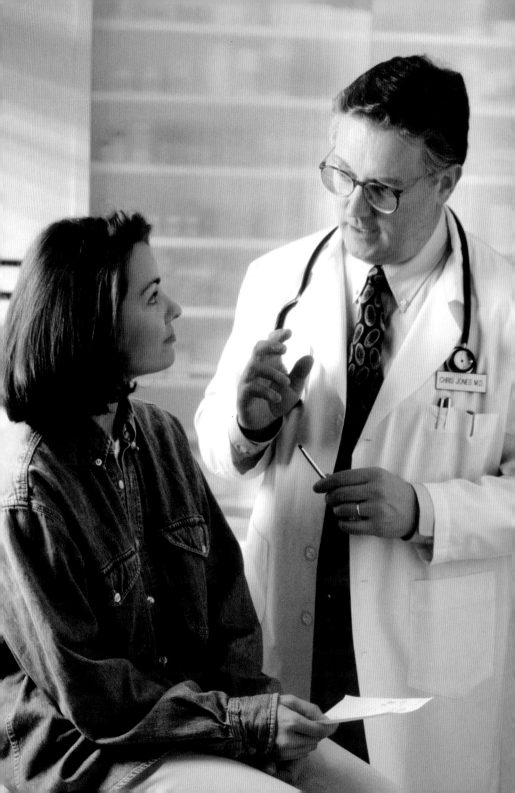

understanding
aging

It is a fact of life that we all age. Our bodies are at their peak at about age 25. Signs of aging start from about age 30, as our skin begins to sag and our short-term memory starts to decline. Between ages 50 and 60, our brains start shrinking, our hearing and sight worsen, our joints stiffen, and our heart and lungs become less efficient. However, illness, loss of mobility, and a decline in mental ability are not inevitable as we age. Many factors affect aging, and we can stay fit and active for 80 years or more. This section will identify what you can change in your life to help "beat the years" and advise you when to seek professional help.

why do we age?

No one knows exactly why we age. Many theories have been put forward, but scientists cannot agree on a universal theory for aging. However, most antiaging experts do agree that it is probably due to a combination of the genes we inherit, the lifestyles we lead, the environment we live in, and our mental attitudes about life and aging itself. At present, we can do little to influence our genetic makeup, although scientific breakthroughs in this field may be only a few decades away. However, there is a lot we can do to change our lifestyles and environment.

Biological theories for aging

Scientists have proposed several different theories about aging. The first theory is that we have genes that cause our body to age. Scientists now believe that the genetic processes associated with aging are far less complex than previously thought. It seems that only a relatively small number of the thousands of genes we have are involved in the aging process.

The ongoing human genome project, which is mapping every human gene, has thrown some light on this subject and much is hoped for in the future. This project should allow us to better understand the genetics of aging, as well as provide information on diseases that are inherited or genetically influenced.

Scientists have also come to believe that it is not so much that our bodies age but that different organs age at different rates. Therefore the human body is as weak as its weakest part. Someone might die earlier than expected because one organ, say the heart, stops working, even though the rest of their body is fine. The advent of organ transplants—such as heart transplants, which are now routine—is one medical breakthrough that can help people live longer, healthier lives.

Other biological reasons for aging are thought to include:

• increased levels of two aging hormones, insulin (a hormone produced by the pancreas to help the body use glucose) and cortisol (a natural steroid hormone produced by stress).

• decreased levels of those hormones thought to prevent aging, such as the female sex hormones, estrogen and progesterone; the male sex hormone, testosterone; melatonin (a hormone produced by the pineal gland in the brain); and human growth hormone.

• too many destructive free radicals in the body (see antioxidants on p.58).

• a dwindling away of the "biological clocks" (known as telomeres) we have in all our cells, which affect the rate of cell division and are controlled by the enzyme telomerase.

What is aging?

Current thinking proposes that there is "normal" aging, which is the "to be expected" changes that occur in bodily functions as we get older, and there is "pathological" aging. The "normal" changes that occur when we age, such as loss of bone mass and thinning of the skin, do not necessarily cause disease, and "normal" aging does not equate with illness.

A chronic condition, such as osteoarthritis or diabetes, can age people much faster than "normal"; this is sometimes known as "pathological" aging. On average, we all start showing signs of aging at about age 30, when the functioning of most of the body systems begins to decline, but there is no fixed timescale to aging. Lifestyle and genetic factors also influence the process.

We all age at different rates, and by the time we are around age 65, there is much more diversity between us in terms of our health and fitness than when we are in our teens. General factors, as well as our genes, predetermine how fast we age, such as sex, ethnic group, environmental influences, levels of sun exposure, and lifestyle choices such as drinking, smoking, and nutrition.

identifying
your aims

Slowing down the aging process can mean different things to different people. For some, it may be about wanting to live longer, or wanting to look young and beautiful for as long as possible. For others, it may be about wanting to stay healthy and fit throughout life, or staying sexually potent for longer. It is important to identify what your goals are, because this will help you recognize the sort of changes you need to make to help you reach your goals. How you age is up to you, and only you can develop the positive attitudes, practices, and habits that will help you to have the quality of life you want for your entire life.

Setting your goals

If you want to have a wrinkle-free face at age 50, then stopping smoking, avoiding the sun, doing daily face exercises, and taking certain vitamin and mineral supplements might be the best choices for you. If you want to be fit, mobile, and healthy well into old age, then yoga or tai chi might be suitable activities. If you want greater longevity, then stopping smoking, eating a healthy diet, and keeping slim and fit will help to reduce your risk of heart disease and should increase your life expectancy. If you want to remain sexual potent for longer, hormone replacement therapy (if you are female) or testosterone replacement therapy (if you are male) might be the answer. Although hormone replacement therapy does not increase potency, it can affect vaginal conditions, which can indirectly affect libido.

Identifying preventive measures

If you are fit and well now, it is important to try to stay that way by taking preventive measures to look after your body and mind. These measures include eating a healthy diet, exercising regularly, stopping smoking, drinking moderately, and taking time to relax and rest. You should also have regular medical checkups, such as screening for breast, cervical, and testicular cancer; have your blood pressure and blood cholesterol and blood glucose levels monitored; and have annual eye exams. Ways to protect yourself and prevent disease include practicing safe sex, avoiding sunburn, and having good posture. It can also be argued that having a meaningful purpose in life keeps you younger longer. If you already suffer from health problems, certain dietary and lifestyle measures, conventional medicines, and complementary therapies may help you get better. However, if you have a persistent health problem, you should always see your doctor first (see when to see a doctor p.16). When your doctor checks your blood pressure, you should also have a test for diabetes mellitus, an evaluation for cardiovascular changes, and a check of your iron and antioxidant levels.

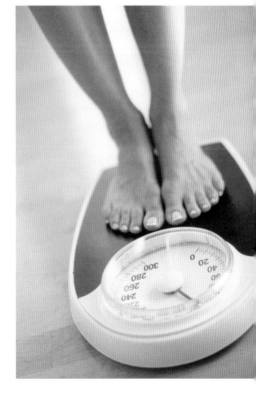

Whatever antiaging measures you take, set realistic goals, and don't try to change too much at once. Address one area of your life at a time that could benefit from changes. If you decide to stop smoking and lose weight, cut out cigarettes first and when you've successfully kicked that habit, turn your attention to losing weight. Scientific evidence shows that it is never to late to try "beating the years."

Maintaining an ideal weight is one way to stay healthy and fit and to look younger longer.

when to see a doctor

It is fine to treat minor ailments such as colds, hay fever, mild tension headaches, indigestion, and mild aches and pains yourself. However, if you have a condition that persists for more than a week or if you suffer from a chronic disease, you should seek professional help. This includes such conditions as asthma, epilepsy, heart disease, diabetes, cancer, stomach ulcers, inflammatory bowel diseases, and severe depression.

Illness, disease and your symptoms

It is important to recognize that *illness* and *disease* are not the same. An illness is what you, the patient, experiences. A disease is what a doctor diagnoses, based on your signs and symptoms. For example, you might suffer from wheezing and a cough, which your doctor diagnoses as asthma and treats accordingly. Sometimes, however, you may feel ill but your doctor might not recognize your symptoms as a diagnosable disease. This does not mean that nothing is wrong with you. It could be that conventional medicine just doesn't have a diagnosis to fit what you have yet. Such symptoms are sometimes called "medically unexplained symptoms."

Many conventional doctors find it hard to treat illnesses that do not fit a diagnosable disease—and this is where complementary medicine comes into its own. Those therapies with their own traditional systems of medicine (such as Chinese herbalism, acupuncture, Ayurveda, and homeopathy) tend to base their diagnosis on

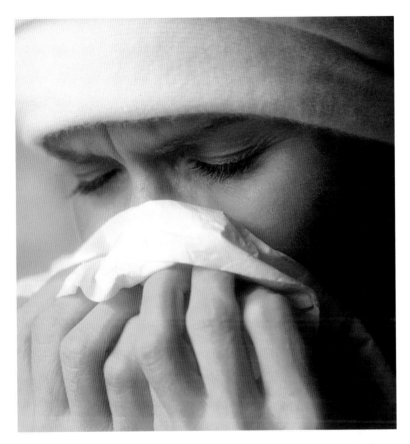

Cold viruses are rapidly spread by sneezing. The common cold usually clears up in a week or two, without needing any medical treatment.

the symptoms the patient describes and on what they can see, feel, hear, and smell. They then fit the treatment to the patient, rather than try to treat a diagnosed disease.

Illness and aging

Although many people stay fit and healthy well into their later years, some develop chronic diseases associated with aging, such as heart problems, diabetes, arthritis, or osteoporosis. A chronic health problem can age people much faster than

PROBLEMS REQUIRING IMMEDIATE ATTENTION

The following is a list of the major warning signs and symptoms of serious illness. If you experience any of these, you should seek professional help. If you have any persistent, recurrent, or unexplained health problem or your signs or symptoms worsen, you again need to consult your doctor.

- *Chest pain or discomfort*
- *Unusual shortness of breath*
- *Unexplained dizziness*
- *Persistent cough, sore throat, or hoarseness*
- *Coughing up blood*
- *Difficulty in swallowing*
- *Mouth ulceration lasting more than a month*
- *Lasting abdominal pain or indigestion*
- *Vomiting of coffee grounds material or blood*
- *Unexplained changes in bowel or bladder habits*
- *Passing blood, either bright red or black, in the stools*
- *Passing blood in the urine*
- *Change in shape or size of testicle, or a lump or swelling*
- *Vaginal bleeding between periods, after sex, or after menopause*
- *Unusual vaginal discharge*
- *A lump or thickening in a breast, change in shape or size of a breast, discharge or bleeding from a nipple, flattening of a nipple, dimpling or puckering of skin over a breast*
- *Persistent, unexplained weight loss*
- *Long-term, unexplained tiredness*
- *Changes in a mole on the skin. Look for any change in the shape, color, or size. Check using the ABCD guide: asymmetry, border, color, diameter*
- *Any new, unexplained lumps or swellings*
- *Any sore that does not heal*
- *Sudden severe headaches, persistent one-sided headaches, blurred or disturbed vision*
- *Frequent back pain that persists even during rest*
- *Unexplained leg pain and swelling*
- *Excessive thirst*

"normal." However, if you do have a chronic health problem, don't give up hope. You can try many things that, although they may not cure you, can help to relieve your symptoms, increase your life expectancy, and improve your mobility and sense of well-being.

Regular checkups

As you get older, frequent health checkups are very important. Your doctor may be able to preempt certain conditions or at least help to minimize their effects by taking appropriate action, if taken early enough. A physical examination may reveal a disorder that can be treated before it becomes a problem.

Screening tests can indicate disease. The most basic example of this is the measurement of blood pressure. High blood pressure, or hypertension, can be a warning of imminent stroke or heart disease, and preventive action may be taken. Sometimes drug treatment is necessary, but often changes in lifestyle are worthwhile, such as giving up smoking and not drinking excessive amounts of alcohol, exercising more, and eating a sensible diet. These measures may be enough to help reduce the blood pressure to normal levels, thus averting the need for any further medical intervention.

kicking
bad habits

So what can you do if you are dependent on a drug and want to stop taking it? The first step is to recognize that you have a problem and that you need help. Don't set your goals too high, too soon: Just take one day at a time.

Knowing the health risks

Smoking not only greatly increases the risk of getting diseases like lung cancer, other lung conditions, and heart disease, it also increases the chances of dying early. Alcohol is also addictive and, if consumed in large amounts (more than one drink a day for women and two a day for men—one drink is 12 oz of beer, a glass of wine, or $1\frac{1}{2}$ oz of spirits), can cause heart problems and liver damage. Other addictive drugs, legal and illegal, that people can become dependent on include sedatives like the benzodiazepines and barbiturates; opiates like morphine, heroin, methadone, and codeine; amphetamines; cocaine; crack; and caffeine.

Understanding addiction

Use of substances such as nicotine and alcohol can result in physical and psychological dependence. Whenever you give up something you are addicted to, it can result in unpleasant withdrawal signs and symptoms. These can be physical, such as shaking, fits, sweating, or headaches, or they can be psychological, such as cravings or anxiety. Different substances have different characteristic withdrawal signs and symptoms. Although people typically start taking drugs to get high, they soon find that they have to take them to keep from feeling bad because of the withdrawal signs and symptoms. Patients who have legitimate pain and are undermedicated can have similar behavior to drug abusers when seeking more drugs, but the difference is they stop this behavior once their pain is properly treated. This is called pseudoaddiction.

Stopping smoking

Only about 2 in every 100 smokers who try to stop without any help are successful. Counseling and advice can be beneficial, as can self-help groups. Using nicotine replacement therapy (NRT) or the controversial drug bupropion (Zyban) can roughly double your chances of success, if you also get counseling at the same time. NRT works by giving you nicotine in fixed doses, without the harmful chemicals found in tobacco smoke. It is available as chewing gum, skin patches, lozenges, tablets, nasal spray, or inhaler. Although NRT has some adverse effects (such as feeling or being sick, headache, dizziness, or a racing heartbeat), these are rare. NRT products can also irritate the parts of the body they come into contact with, such as the nose with a nasal spray or skin with a patch.

Bupropion is believed to work on the parts of the brain involved in nicotine addiction. A relatively new drug, it is available only by prescription. Adverse effects include difficulty sleeping and dry mouth, and it also causes fits in certain people. So far, research suggests that acupuncture and hypnotherapy might only be of marginal benefit in helping people give up smoking.

Eliminating other drug problems

Conventional treatments for drug problems include medicines to treat withdrawal symptoms, such as acamprosate (Campral) for alcohol dependence; to make using alcohol an unpleasant experience, such as disulfiram (Antabuse) for alcohol dependence; or to substitute the problem drug with another similar but weaker drug, such as methadone for heroin. Usually, counseling is recommended and an antidepressant prescribed. In severe cases, people with a drug problem need to be treated in hospital or may undergo rehabilitation in a residential setting.

Many complementary therapies are used for drug withdrawal. Whole-body acupuncture and ear acupuncture are probably the most widely accepted and well-researched therapies for alcohol, heroin, cocaine, and crack addiction and are available in many conventional settings. Psychotherapy and counseling are widely used and well-researched. Because alcohol addiction can cause malnourishment, some vitamins and minerals may help people with this dependency. Other therapies, which probably work by promoting relaxation and have quite good evidence to support them, include massage, biofeedback, and yoga.

heart and
circulatory
diseases

About one in every four deaths is due to heart disease caused by blocked coronary (heart) arteries, a condition known as atherosclerosis, which stems from high blood cholesterol levels. Two big factors in heart disease are how you live your life and what you eat.

Common signs

If you develop heart disease, you are at increased risk for developing angina (chest pain from the heart not getting enough oxygen), a heart attack (see p.24), an arrhythmia (an abnormal heartbeat, which can cause breathlessness, dizziness, or even death), or heart failure (when the heart cannot pump effectively, leading to breathlessness, tiredness, swollen ankles, and eventually a shortened life expectancy).

Atherosclerosis can also occur in arteries in other parts of the body, such as the brain, kidneys, or legs. This can lead to strokes, kidney failure, or poor circulation in the legs, which may necessitate even amputation. Other problems of the heart and circulatory system include high cholesterol levels, high blood pressure, heart attacks, diabetes, and chilblains.

Most heart problems can be avoided or improved significantly by taking appropriate action. To reduce your risk of heart disease, you should eat a healthy diet (see nutrition and healthy eating, p.54), reduce your sodium intake, avoid smoking tobacco, drink only the recommended amount of alcohol, exercise regularly (see p.64), lose excess weight, and reduce your stress levels (see p.78).

High cholesterol levels

Cholesterol is a type of fat that your body makes and that you can get from your diet. It comes in different types. Low-density lipoprotein (LDL) cholesterol is "bad cholesterol" because it "dumps" cholesterol in your arteries, and the more you have, the more likely you are to develop atherosclerosis. High-density lipoprotein (HDL) cholesterol is "good, or protective, cholesterol" because it "mops" up cholesterol in the body, and the more you have, the less likely you are to have atherosclerosis. If you have high cholesterol levels, you may need to take a cholesterol-lowering drug, such as a statin. Reducing the amount of cholesterol in your diet can also help, but more important, you need to cut down on the amount of full-fat dairy products, fried foods, and saturated animal fats, because the liver converts these to LDL cholesterol. Replacing saturated fats in your diet with healthier fats can help to lower cholesterol levels. Healthier fats include polyunsaturated fats found, for example, in oily fish like sardines, herring, and mackerel; cold-pressed vegetable fats; essential fatty acids; and monounsaturated fats such as olive oil and rapeseed oil. Oat bran can also be beneficial, because it contains a lot of soluble fiber, which has been shown to help lower blood cholesterol levels, although it is probably only helpful in the context of a healthy diet. Certain herbs are also thought to be beneficial. Strong evidence also shows that psyllium, garlic, and guar gum can all help to reduce blood cholesterol levels and so may lower your risk of heart disease.

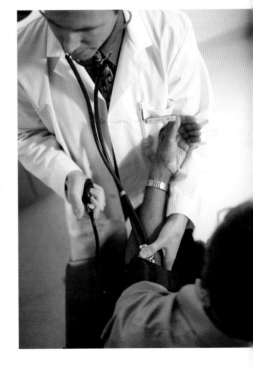

Blood pressure can be measured quickly and easily by a doctor, and is a prime indicator for heart disease. There are many medical and complementary treatments, and lifestyle changes, that can help lower blood pressure.

Other popular options to lower cholesterol levels include:

Exercise—increases levels of HDL (good) cholesterol

Weight loss—increases insulin sensitivity, which allows insulin levels to fall, thus reducing a powerful risk factor for coronary artery disease (CAD)

Niacin—a B vitamin that promotes more effective carbohydrate metabolism

Garlic—shown in some studies to lower cholesterol levels

Gugul lipid—an Ayurvedic herb with minimal adverse effects

Policasamine—a plant extract that reduces cholesterol with minimal adverse effects

High blood pressure

High blood pressure, or hypertension, can cause or worsen heart disease because it can damage arteries and put a strain on your heart. Conventional treatments include several different types of drugs such as beta-blockers (e.g., atenolol), angiotensin-converting enzyme inhibitors (e.g., enalapril), diuretics (e.g., sodium bendroflumethiazide), and calcium antagonists (e.g., nifedipine). Reducing the amount of salt in your diet, losing excess weight, exercising regularly, and reducing stress levels (see p.78) will all help. Other popular options include taking extra magnesium, which can improve dilation of blood vessels, and essential fatty acids, which can reduce the quantity of arachidonic acid that is converted into inflammatory compounds called cytokines, which promote CAD.

Although high blood pressure can be a sign of heart, liver, or kidney disease, often it has no obvious cause, in which case complementary medicine can be helpful when used with—or in mild hypertension, it can be used instead of—conventional drugs. There is good evidence that hawthorn berries can lower blood pressure, help to improve the circulation of blood in the heart, make the heart's pumping action more efficient. Ju hua (chrysanthemum flowers) may help by relaxing the heart and improving blood flow, but more research is needed to confirm this. Acupuncture, autogenic training, and meditation may also be beneficial.

Heart attack

A heart attack (myocardial infarction) occurs when part of the heart muscle dies after its normal blood supply has been blocked. Usually, it is due to a blood clot in one of the coronary arteries surrounding the heart. In most cases, the artery is already narrowed because of fatty deposits (atherosclerosis). Research has also found that around 50 percent of people have blood that is more prone to clotting than others, meaning it is hypercoagulable. Signs and symptoms of a heart attack include pain across the center of the chest; pain spreading to the arms, neck, or jaw; sweating; feeling or being sick; a racing heartbeat; pallor; breathlessness; and collapse.

You are at increased risk for a heart attack if you have a family history of heart disease, or if you smoke, have high blood pressure or high cholesterol levels, are overweight, have diabetes, or drink too much alcohol. Your risk increases as you get older. If you have a heart attack, you can reduce your risk of having another one by exercising regularly, eating a healthy diet (see nutrition and healthy eating, p.54), and stopping smoking. Conventional treatment usually includes morphine for pain relief, with a clot-busting drug. Your doctor will probably also suggest that you take a low dose of aspirin every day to help prevent another attack and may prescribe other drugs to lower your blood pressure or cholesterol levels. Complementary therapies that may help after a heart attack include tai chi, naturopathy, relaxation, breathing exercises, and meditation.

Varicose veins

Varicose veins are blue swollen veins just beneath the skin surface. They are most common in the lower legs and are more common in women than men. They are due to weak valves in the veins that lead to pooling of blood in the extremities. Factors that contribute to varicose veins are family history, diet and lifestyle, constipation, obesity, pregnancy, standing for long periods, and lack of exercise. Conventional treatment involves wearing support tights, exercising, resting with the legs raised above the level of the heart, injecting chemicals to collapse the veins, or surgery.

Not much scientific evidence supports using complementary therapies to treat varicose veins, except certain herbs such as horse chestnut (strong evidence), gotu kola (moderate evidence), and butcher's broom (some evidence). Moderate evidence also supports using hydrotherapy, yoga (especially inverted postures such as headstand), or aromatherapy with oils such as cypress that are said to tone the blood vessels.

Chilblains

Chilblains are itchy, reddish blue swellings on the fingers and toes caused by the cold, poor circulation in the feet, a lack of exercise, and a poor diet. Squeezing

The heart

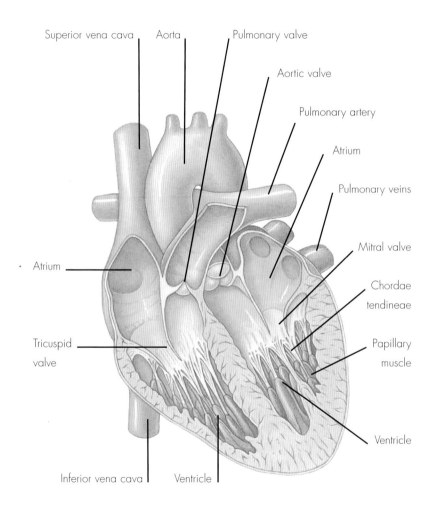

Superior vena cava   Aorta   Pulmonary valve

Aortic valve

Pulmonary artery

Atrium

Pulmonary veins

Mitral valve

Chordae tendineae

Papillary muscle

Atrium

Tricuspid valve

Ventricle

Inferior vena cava   Ventricle

Oxygenated blood from the lungs enters the left atrium of the heart, passes to the left ventricle, and circulates to the rest of the body. Used, or deoxygenated, blood from the body enters the right atrium, passes into the right ventricle, and then returns to the lungs to pick up fresh oxygen.

the juice of a piece of fresh gingerroot over an unopened chilblain might help. Taking garlic regularly can improve circulation, as can regular massage.

Help with losing weight

The most effective way to lose excess weight is to reduce the amount of calories you eat and to exercise regularly. To keep weight off, you need to eat a healthy low-fat, low-calorie diet, and exercise. Most dieters who concentrate only on reducing their calorie intake, tend to put back any weight they have lost within 2 to 3 years. Talking with a dietitian or counselor, or attending a weight loss group might help you to change your eating habits.

About one-third of the population has some resistance to insulin. Typically, these people have abdominal obesity, hypertension, low HDL levels, and high triglyceride levels, leading to high levels of insulin. This causes the so-called Syndrome X or Metabolic Syndrome. Starchy foods such as bread, pasta, white rice and potatoes are turned into sugar in the stomach and absorbed rapidly into the bloodstream. People who are insulin resistant must make larger amounts of it to control blood sugar levels. This insulin resistance causes the liver to produce LDL, the "bad" cholesterol, and raises stress hormone levels. It also makes the body store fat, thus contributing to obesity, which increases blood pressure and the risk of heart attack and stroke. The solution is to limit the intake of carbohydrates, and take exercise.

Medical methods

If you are obese or have a serious health problem because of your weight, and diet and exercise haven't worked, your doctor might as a last resort prescribe a drug such as orlistat (Xenical), which works by stopping enzymes in your stomach from breaking down fat, so less fat is absorbed into your system. Another drug, sibutramine (Reductil) affects the appetite control centers in the brain. Methylcellulose (Citrucel), which is commonly used as a laxative for constipation, is sometimes used because it swells in the digestive system and produces a feeling of fullness, but this is not proven. Finally, the appetite suppressant phentermine (Ionamin) is sometimes used in specialist clinics along with treatments such as counseling; however, these drugs have serious side effects and can be addictive. The supplement chitosan, from the shells of shellfish, with various fungi is supposed to bind to fat, preventing it from being absorbed, but this is not proven, and study results of its effectiveness for weight loss are mixed.

diabetes

This is a serious condition where the body has problems controlling the level of sugar in the blood. The full name for the disease is diabetes mellitus and there are two variants.

Type 1 diabetes, also known as early-onset or juvenile diabetes, occurs when the pancreas suddenly stops making insulin. Insulin is a hormone that helps transfer glucose from the bloodstream to cells, where it is used to make energy. This type of diabetes tends to occur first in young people and must be treated with insulin injections. In Type 2, or adult-onset diabetes, which develops more slowly, the pancreas releases increased amounts of insulin into the bloodstream, but not enough to prevent a build-up of sugar in the circulation. This is because this insulin is weak, and insufficent to keep blood sugar levels within the normal range. Thus insulin sensitivity is reduced, and insulin resistance develops. Type 2 diabetes is more common after 40 years of age and it is this type we are concerned with.

What causes type 2 diabetes?

The biggest cause of type 2 diabetes seems to be being overweight. In the West, as the incidence of obesity increases, so does the incidence of type 2 diabetes. Stress and a lack of exercise are also factors. It is also more common in Asians and Afro Caribbeans and there might be a family tendency to the disease. The best way to avoid diabetes is to maintain a healthy weight, take regular exercise, and to eat a low-carbohydrate diet. It has been the accepted wisdom that foods with a low glycemic index will best prevent the onset of diabetes, but guidelines issued recently by the American Diabetic Association suggest that the glycemic index of your food is not as important as controlling the total amount of carbohydrate you eat.

How is type 2 diabetes treated?

People with type 2 diabetes don't usually need to inject insulin. Dietary changes alone might be enough to start with, such as cutting down the amount of sugary foods eaten and increasing the amount of starchy foods in the diet, as these help to slow down the absorption of sugar into the body. It is also important to lose any excess weight. If dietary measures are not enough, then conventional treatment consists of drugs to help keep blood glucose levels normal, such as metformin, a sulfonylurea, or a glitazone. In time, a combination of drugs might be needed. Eventually, some people with type 2 diabetes need insulin injections.

There are also some complementary therapies that might be beneficial in type 2 diabetes. The herbs fenugreek seeds, goat's rue, garlic, and guar gum might help to reduce blood sugar levels but should not be used without professional advice. There is also tentative evidence that evening primrose oil can help in people with diabetic neuropathy, and that yoga may enhance the function of the pancreas and help to reduce stress. Naturopathy might help by recommending a low sugar and high fibre diet, with the addition of oats to stabilize sugar levels and chromium to help normalize blood sugar breakdown.

If you think you may have developed diabetes, it is vital to seek professional help. If you have diabetes, it is important to have regular health check-ups, as it is associated with several long-term problems such as kidney, eye, nerve, and skin damage. People with diabetes are more likely to develop heart disease; their risk of dying from a heart attack is two to three times that of a non-diabetic.

COMMON SYMPTOMS OF DIABETES

Many older people with type 2 diabetes only become aware that they have the disease when they go for a routine blood or urine test, even though they may have symptoms. Common ones include:

- excessive thirst
- frequent urination
- tiredness
- weakness
- numbness or tingling in the hands and feet
- blurred vision
- impotence in men

back
pain

Back pain is the second most common health complaint after the common cold. It is responsible for millions of lost working days each year, and nearly all of us will suffer from back pain at least once in our lifetime. The older we get, the more likely we are to experience back pain, as the years of wear and tear on our back accumulate. However, it is never too late to do something to help prevent back problems or to stop them from recurring. Back pain may be constant or unpredictable, it may only occur when you do a specific thing such as walking, or it may be a dull ache or a sharp, stabbing pain.

Understanding the causes

Overall, the most common cause of back pain is poor posture, such as slouching, or awkward movements, such as stretching and twisting to reach something. Some people are more prone to it: Back pain is more common in tall people with long spines, overweight people, and men. Usually, no actual pathological change can be found, in which case the doctor may then refer to the pain as "nonspecific," "mechanical," or "idiopathic," meaning that the cause is unknown. Typically, this type of back pain is felt as discomfort across the lower back or over the lower spine, and it recurs periodically in the same form. The pain might also radiate into the buttocks or legs and is associated with stiffness first thing in the morning. Movement eases this type of pain and staying in the same position for any length of time aggravates it.

X rays of older people nearly always show osteoarthritis, though it typically does not cause pain. Lower back pain is commonly caused by nerve impingement in the spine or ligament laxity, which puts undue stress on the joints of the spine. Occasionally, back pain is due to a serious underlying disorder, such as cancer, a ruptured disc, or osteoporotic fracture. If you have back pain that gets worse, if it is constant whatever you do, or if you have weakness, numbness, or tingling in a leg, difficulty in passing urine or stools, or any other symptoms or pain elsewhere in your body, then you should consult your doctor to make sure the pain is not due to a serious underlying neurological problem.

Treating nonspecific back pain

The best treatment for nonspecific back pain is to maintain your normal daily activities as much as possible, even taking a mild painkiller such as acetaminophen, aspirin, or ibuprofen for a few days to help you do so. If the pain then persists for more than a few days, a course of chiropractic manipulation or osteopathy is definitely worth trying, but this treatment will be less effective for chronic pain that has lasted more than about 3 months.

Acupuncture (see p.100) is probably more effective in such cases. Alternatively, you could try physiotherapy or massage. Regular exercise is also a good idea. It can strengthen the back and trunk muscles, which stabilizes the back, and can

Back pain may be due to poor posture, weak abdominal muscles, or muscle injury. Manipulation or massage may help to relieve the pain.

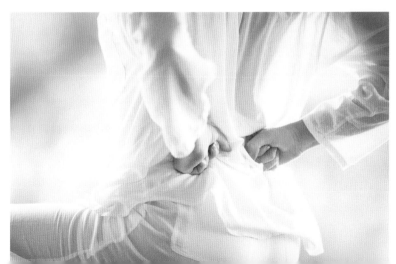

prevent problems. What's more, it can help you lose weight. However, certain movements and activities can put a strain on the back and aggravate an existing problem. If you have a back problem, it is best, at least initially, to consult an experienced and well-trained teacher or therapist. As far as aerobic exercise is concerned, walking is an excellent choice, as long as you wear well-fitting shoes with cushioned rubber soles to prevent jarring. Cycling and swimming are also good, but if you do the breaststroke, don't keep your head out of water all the time because doing so can strain your neck. Make sure you stop if you feel any pain, and remember to tell your exercise instructor or teacher about your condition. Sports that are best avoided by people with "bad" backs are gymnastics, judo, rowing, squash, tennis, weight lifting, wrestling, and other contact sports.

Tips for easing back pain

If your posture is a major cause of your back pain, then yoga (see p.114) or the Alexander technique (see p.74) might be the answer. You could also try herbal medicine. Pain due to muscle tension may respond to cramp bark or valerian; back pain due to osteoarthritis, devil's claw; and chronic back pain, willow. St. John's wort can help to relieve the mild depression often associated with chronic back pain. You can also try these other helpful tips: Always sleep on a firm mattress or place a board under your mattress; if you have to spend hours sitting down, get up every 20–30 minutes to stretch and move around; and, if stress is causing your back muscles to tighten, then try a relaxation technique (see p.82).

Prolotherapy

Prolotherpy is gaining ground as an alternative to surgery for some injuries. It involves a series of injections of simple substances such as sugar, often combined with a local anesthetic, into damaged tissues. These substances act as local irritants, stimulating the tissue to proliferate, growing new tissue to repair the damaged tissue.

Clinical results from doctors who use prolotherapy suggest that it can be used to treat various problems. These include ligament laxity in the knee or ankle, tennis elbow or golfer's elbow, Achilles tendon injuries, and lower back pain.

Self-help with simple back twists

The standing twist and the sitting twist are two simple yoga postures that can prove invaluable for anyone suffering from back pain. Perform them slowly and carefully, but do not force your body into the position if you feel uncomfortable or excessive strain, because this could lead to injury. The aim is to stretch and tone the muscles. If repeated regularly, the postures help the body to become stronger and more supple. These postures can be practiced anytime and are good to do at work, particularly if you have to sit for long hours. All you will need is an upright chair with a fixed back.

Standing twist (maricyasana)

Take a chair and place it sideways against a wall. Stand in front of it with your legs gently against it and straight. Raise the leg nearest the wall and place its foot flat on the chair seat. Keep the other leg straight and firm. Put your hands on your hips and stretch your back upward. Then turn your trunk so it is facing the wall and turn your head farther so you are looking over the shoulder nearest the wall. Bring your hands up to shoulder level and, with your elbows slightly bent, press your hands against the wall to help you turn more. Every two or three breaths, try and turn more; as you breathe in, try and stretch your back up more, and as you breathe out, try and turn a little more. Stay for 20–30 seconds. Then exhale and turn to face the chair again, bringing the raised leg down. Turn the chair around, and repeat on the other side. Finally, repeat on both sides once or twice again.

Sitting twist (bharadvajasana)

Sit sideways on a chair with your buttocks and most of your thighs on the chair, your knees together, and your feet flat on the floor. Sit up straight. Turn to face the back of the chair, turning the hips as much as possible at first, followed by the waist, chest, and shoulders. Place your hands at either end of the top of the chair back. If you are seated with your left side against the chair back, push with your left hand and pull with your right hand to help you turn more. You are aiming to eventually have your chest parallel to the chair back. When you have turned as much as you can, turn your head to look over your left shoulder. Hold this position for 20–30 seconds, breathing evenly, then exhale and turn to the front. Get up, turn to sit down on the other side, and repeat. Finally, repeat on both sides once or twice again.

arthritic

conditions

There are over 100 rheumatic diseases. Although many are extremely rare, osteoarthritis—the most common rheumatic disease—affects most of us in old age and can result in pain, swelling, and stiffness in one or more joints.

Understanding arthritis

Arthritis is a disease where the cartilage surfaces inside a joint wear down. It tends to develop gradually as we age. Most people have osteoarthritis in at least one joint by the time they are in their sixties, the most commonly affected ones being the knees, hips, and joints at the base of the neck and lower back. Your risk of osteoarthritis is increased if you are overweight, if you overuse a joint by playing a particular sport, or if you had a serious or recurrent injury to a joint when you were younger.

Rheumatoid arthritis is a severe rheumatic disease that can affect the whole body. The cause is unknown, but it is thought to be an autoimmune disease, where the body seems to attack itself. It can result in pain, stiffness, swelling, tenderness, warmth, and redness in several joints at once. Other signs and symptoms include general weakness and debility, fever, and loss of grip strength in the hands. The disease flares up and dies down intermittently, but when the joints flare up, there can be lasting damage that can eventually lead to immobility and deformity of the affected joints. Rheumatoid arthritis usually first affects people in their thirties.

Treating arthritic problems

Conventional medicine has no cure for any arthritic disorder. Treatment of osteoarthritis usually includes painkillers such as acetaminophen or nonsteroidal anti-inflammatory drugs (NSAIDs). (These drugs can have severe and potentially life-threatening consequences, such as kidney failure and liver disease.) You might also given exercises to do to by a physiotherapist to strengthen the muscles around your arthritic joint. If a joint becomes very painful or stiff, you may be referred for surgery to have the joint replaced. In the past, conventional treatment for early rheumatoid arthritis was similar to that for osteoarthritis. Now, however, in an attempt to slow disease progression and prevent lasting damage, it usually starts with a disease-modifying antirheumatic drug such as methotrexate or penicillamine.

Many people with rheumatic problems also use complementary therapies, partly because conventional medicine is not always successful and partly because the conventional drugs used to treat them have some adverse effects. Acupuncture is widely used for rheumatic disorders, and evidence shows that it is beneficial.

Naturopathy, or nutritional therapy, can also help, because certain foods, such as citrus fruits and caffeine, tend to aggravate rheumatic problems. Evidence shows that the supplements glucosamine and chondroitin relieve joint pain and that fish oils relieve inflammation. Several western herbs have recently been shown to be as effective as NSAIDs, but without the side effects. Devil's claw has been shown in clinical trials to help relieve the pain of osteoarthritis, and willow helps to relieve chronic pain. Meadowsweet, cramp bark, nettle leaf, or feverfew may help, but this needs confirming. Guggul is thought to be the best Ayurvedic medicine for arthritic conditions, whereas frankincense has been shown to help in rheumatoid arthritis and—along with winter cherry, turmeric, and minerals—osteoarthritis. Asafoetida paste is used externally on painful joints, and neem is used to reduce inflammation. In Chinese medicine, the herbs gentian, Chinese quince, and clematis are used for rheumatic problems.

Self-help for short-term relief of joint pains

Celery seeds can ease painful and stiff joints, but you may need to take them for some weeks before seeing results. If a joint is hot and swollen, place a pack of frozen peas on it to cool it and reduce the pain. Lavender oil (10 drops in one teaspoon of almond oil) massaged into the joint can bring relief. If a joint is cold, soak in a hot bath with 5 drops of rosemary oil added to it, or apply a hot cabbage leaf. An Epsom salt bath can bring relief. Fill your bathtub halfway with warm water, add two handfuls of Epsom salts (magnesium sulphate), and soak for 10–20 minutes, topping off with hot water to keep warm. Dry without rinsing off the salts.

osteoporosis

In osteoporosis, bones lose mass and density, becoming brittle, fragile, and more likely to break, even after a minor fall. Almost everyone's bones become less dense as they get older because the body becomes less efficient at absorbing and using calcium, which is a vital component of bone. When a person's bone density falls below a certain level, they are said to have osteoporosis.

Understanding osteoporosis

A woman's risk of osteoporosis increases dramatically during and after the menopause because the fall in estrogen levels during this time causes bone loss to accelerate; estrogen helps the body to absorb and use calcium. Men tend not to be affected until in their seventies. Taking oral corticosteroids, particularly for a long time, can also cause osteoporosis. Other risk factors include smoking, excessive alcohol and caffeine intake, a sedentary lifestyle, a diet low in calcium, low exposure to sunlight, family history, and being white or Asian. Osteoporosis is hard to detect and is usually discovered after a bone has broken. Reduced bone density can be screened using X-ray densiometry. Biochemical urine tests can be done, but they have limitations and are expensive. The bones most likely to be affected by osteoporosis are the spine, hip, and wrist bones. If left untreated, osteoporosis can lead to collapsing of the bones in the spine, which can cause pain, disability, and significant loss of height.

Preventing and treating osteoporosis

The best way to prevent osteoporosis is to make sure you have enough calcium and vitamin D in your diet. Dairy products like milk and cheese are an important source of calcium. Low-fat and nonfat milk and other low-fat dairy products are good choices because they are a good source of minerals and they are low in fat. Other good sources are tofu, sardines, watercress, dried figs, almonds, dried apricots, green leafy vegetables, and oatmeal. It may be a good idea for

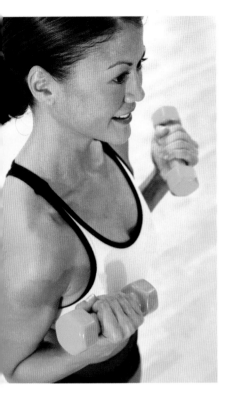

Regular weight training can help to increase bone density.

postmenopausal women to take a calcium supplement. Vitamin K, magnesium, boron, possibly silica, and other trace elements may also help. Sunlight is important, because the body needs it to make vitamin D, so older people who are housebound are at risk for osteoporosis because they rarely go outside. Weight-bearing exercises (such as weight lifting, walking, and running) also increase bone density for as long as you keep doing them, so it is important to exercise regularly throughout your life.

In conventional medicine, osteoporosis is prevented and treated with drugs that increase bone mass. Hormone replacement therapy may be given—and it does treat osteoporosis—although there is no evidence that it lowers the incidence of fractures beyond age 60. Other drugs include raloxifene, calcitonin, and bisphosphonates such as alendronic acid. Exercise is limited to how severe your condition is and how much pain you're in. Don't do too much too quickly, and stop if you feel any pain. People with severe osteoporosis should try to prevent falls and wear a hip protector, to reduce the risk of hip fractures after a fall. Nutritional therapy advises eating foods high in calcium, little data exists on the effects of complementary therapies on osteoporosis. Herbs that may help include those rich in calcium (such as parsley, sesame seeds, nettle, horsetail, and dandelion leaf) and those that may have a hormonal action (such as sage, black cohosh, and wild yam). Tai chi and yoga may help by increasing strength, flexibility, and balance, which may help prevent falls. It is claimed that homeopathic treatment can reduces bone loss, but this is unproven.

menopause

The word *menopause* means the stopping of the monthly
period (menses) and is a normal stage in a woman's life.
Usually, it takes place between the ages 45 and 55, but
it can happen as early as age 35.

What happens during the menopause?

When a baby girl is born, she has all the eggs in her ovaries that she is going to
have. Eventually, these run out and the ovaries stop releasing eggs. During this time,
the levels of the female sex hormones, estrogen and progesterone, which are
produced by the ovaries, become erratic and fall off. It is the reduction of estrogen
that causes the classical symptoms of the menopause: hot flushes, night sweats,
vaginal dryness, insomnia, depression, and loss of bone density (see osteoporosis
p.36). Many women have no symptoms during their menopausal years, but for
about a third of women, there are unpleasant physical and psychological symptoms.
If you bleed after your periods have stopped, see a doctor.

What treatments are there?

The conventional medical treatment for menopausal symptoms is hormone
replacement therapy (HRT). Women who still have a womb have to take a
combination of a synthetic estrogen and a progestogen (progesterone-like drug)
because estrogen alone increases the risk of endometrial (womb lining) cancer, and
breast and ovarian cancer. Women who have had a hysterectomy only need to take
estrogen. HRT can alleviate symptoms such as hot flushes about 90 per cent of the
time, although only about 20 per cent of women with symptoms choose to take it.

Estrogen and progesterone were thought to have a protective effect against
heart disease (and premenopausal women do have a lower risk of heart disease),
but HRT is no longer given to women to protect against heart disease. It is now
believed that HRT can increase the risk of heart disease during the first year of taking
the medication, or for those already with heart disease. HRT is also unsuitable for

some women, such as those with a history of thrombosis (blood clots) or those with abnormal vaginal bleeding. Some women stop taking HRT because of minor but unpleasant side effects, such as breast tenderness, weight gain, nausea, headaches, itchy skin rashes, and fluid retention. Other conventional drugs used in the menopause are clonidine for severe hot flushes and anti-depressants.

Complementary treatments can also help with menopausal symptoms. There is scientific evidence for naturopathy, nutritional therapy, relaxation techniques, and herbalism. Helpful herbal medicines include St John's wort for mild to moderate depression, valerian for sleeplessness, vervain for stress, and black cohosh, chaste tree, sage, or wild yam for hormonal irregularity. The evidence for black cohosh is particularly strong, followed by that for chaste tree. Vitamin E or pot marigold cream may help with vaginal dryness. Shatavari is an Ayurvedic tonic said to have a regenerative action on the female organs and to contain female hormones that help with symptoms such as dryness, excessive thirst, hot flushes, and loss of libido, although clinical studies are lacking. Therapies such as acupuncture and homeopathy might help, but the evidence is anecdotal.

Counselling or psychotherapy can help depressed women who find it hard to face children leaving home, retirement or ageing. The preventative measures discussed in the sections on heart disease (see p.22) and osteoporosis (see p.36) are also relevant. Natural progesterone creams are promoted to treat menopausal symptoms. One study suggests they might help with hot flushes but there is only limited evidence that they prevent osteoporosis. There is some evidence for the benefits of soy supplements, which contain phytoestrogens with hormonal properties.

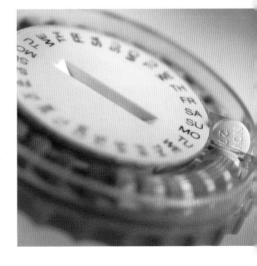

HRT is prescribed for menopausal women to reduce unpleasant symptoms, such as hot flushes, night sweats, insomnia and depression. The incidence of these symptoms varies widely.

prostate
problems

The prostate gland is situated at the base of the bladder and surrounds the urethra, the narrow tube that carries urine and semen to the tip of the penis. The role of the prostate is to produce the fluid that carries sperm. Due to the hormonal changes associated with aging, about one in three men older than age 50 have an enlarged prostate gland caused by benign prostatic hyperplasia (BPH). By the time men are in their seventies, about 70 percent have prostate cancer, although few actually die from the disease. Sometimes, mainly in younger men, the prostate becomes infected (prostatitis) and can be extremely painful.

Knowing the signs and symptoms

When the prostate is swollen, it can press onto the urethra, causing difficulty in passing urine. Possible problems include difficulty in starting to urinate, a thin stream of urine, dribbling after urination, urgency to urinate during the day, and the need to pass urine in the night. Although such signs and symptoms usually are not serious, they should be investigated by a doctor, because they may be indications of prostate cancer.

Preventing prostate problems

Zinc may suppress levels of 5-alpha reductase, which is the enzyme that changes testosterone into a stronger hormone that increases the likelihood of BPH, so a diet rich in zinc might protect against BPH. Particularly good sources of zinc are pumpkin seeds, whole wheat, rye, oats, almonds, peas, oily fish, shellfish, seaweed, asparagus, mushrooms, and lean meat. Men who eat a lot of saturated animal fats are at greatest risk for prostate cancer. A low-fat diet reduces the risk. There may also be a link between prostate cancer and sexually transmitted diseases. Research has not shown whether having a vasectomy increases the risk. Some research suggests that men who play a lot of sports before puberty may reduce their risk of prostate cancer.

Treating prostate problems

Complementary treatments for prostate problems include herbs such as saw palmetto, an anti-inflamatory agent that reduces the size of the prostate, African plum, or nettle root for men with an enlarged prostate gland. Scientific trials have confirmed the effectiveness of saw palmetto in relieving swelling and inflammation of the gland. Saw palmetto is also safe and has been shown to be as effective as conventional drugs. The evidence for other herbs is still tentative. A naturopath would recommend a diet rich in zinc or even zinc supplements, and a common homeopathic remedy for an enlarged prostate is Sabal.

In conventional medicine, the initial treatment for prostate cancer varies. If the cancer is slow growing, which is often the case in men older than age 70, then the usual strategy is to "watch and wait." If treatment is needed, it usually involves either a drug known as a gonadorelin analog, such as buserelin or goserelin, which acts on the sex hormones in the body, or an operation to remove the part of the tumor blocking the urethra. If these measures are unsuccessful, radiotherapy or other drugs might be used, such as an antiandrogen like cyproterone acetate, which suppresses the production of testosterone. Alternatively, the whole prostate gland might be removed surgically through an incision in the abdomen (a total prostatectomy). The nerves that cause erection and sphincter control are commonly injured during prostate surgery, but nerve-sparing laparoscopic procedures are becoming more available. Prostatitis is treated conventionally with bed rest, painkillers, and antibiotics. An enlarged prostate can be treated with surgery to cut away the prostate tissue blocking the urethra. The procedure is usually done by passing a fine tube with a camera and cutting device attached to it along the urethra. Drugs may be used to shrink the prostate. These include finasteride, an alpha reductase inhibitor, and selective alpha-blockers such as prazosin and indoramin. Terazosin and tamsulosin are also commonly used.

sexual
problems

Sexual problems include loss of libido or a reduced sex drive, which can affect both men and women, and impotence, or the inability to attain or maintain an erection (erectile dysfunction). Both can stem from a change in hormone levels; a chronic condition like diabetes, exhaustion, too much alcohol, tobacco smoke, or a drug, either recreational or prescribed. Emotional factors can play a part, such as depression, relationship problems, or stress. Impotence also seems to become increasingly common with age, although there is no reason to view it as an inevitable. Interest in sex and sexual activity can last a lifetime.

Treatments for sexual problems

In conventional medicine, if impotence is suspected to stem from an emotional cause, you might be referred to a sex therapist or counselor. You might also be prescribed a drug such as sildenafil (Viagra) or alprostadil (Muse). These drugs should never be used without the supervision of a doctor, because they can have serious consequences, such as a heart attack, or even death. L-arganine is an amino acid that has been successful in treating impotence and protects circulation to the heart. In severe cases of impotence, a penile implant may be inserted surgically or injections may be given. Testosterone implants are commonly used to treat the loss of libido in women and men, although this can result in masculinizing side effects.

Complementary treatments include herbs to restore the sex drive or treat impotence. Yohimbe bark is a popular herb that comes from central Africa, and there is some evidence that it can help treat impotence. Although no studies have compared it directly with sildenafil, if results from studies of yohimbe versus a placebo are compared with similar studies of sildenafil, the two seem to be similarly effective for impotence. Yohimbe should not be taken by anyone with heart, kidney, or liver disease; anxiety; or high blood pressure; also, it should be used with care in men with certain prostate problems. There is also positive, but less convincing evidence for the benefits of ginkgo biloba and ginseng. Gokshura, taken as a milk decoction, is used in Ayurvedic medicine (see p.123) as a powerful aphrodisiac, and damiana is used as an aphrodisiac in South America.

Low sexual desire, impotence, lower back pain, and poor memory often occur together and Chinese medicine regards them as a weakness in kidney yin and yang qi, so herbs such as he shou wu (see p.124) or gou qi zi (wolfberry) might be used. The Chinese herb we wei zi (schizandra berries) enhances staying power.

In women, hormonal fluctuation during the menstrual cycle or during menopause can also result in loss of libido, and herbs that affect the sex hormones, like chaste tree (see p.39), licorice root, black cohosh, and dong quai can help. The essential oils melissa, ylang-ylang, rose, patchouli, sandalwood, and jasmine are all said to improve sexual performance. Hypnosis may also help if there is a psychological element to your problem, and some weak evidence shows the benefits of acupuncture.

Pelvic floor exercises

Exercising the pubococcygeal muscle at the base of your spine may help you maintain an erection and improve your sexual staying power. This muscle is the one that, if contracted, stops urine in midflow. Perform these exercises daily. Contract the muscle and count to five then relax it. Repeat this cycle as fast as you can about 10 times. Next, bear down on the muscle, just as if you are trying to force urine out, then relax completely.

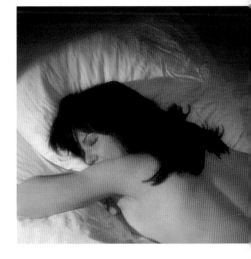

Relaxation and rest are both important to maintain a healthy libido.

memory

loss

Many people believe that their capacity for remembering things diminishes as they get older; however, most people can take certain steps to keep their memories alive and their minds active.

Dementia is not a normal part of aging but a disease characterized by significant mental deterioration—forgetfulness, confusion, behavioral and personality changes, aggression, and disorientation. Stress, insomnia, depression, or even boredom can cause problems with our memory at any age.

Understanding Alzheimer's disease

The most common form of dementia is Alzheimer's disease, which affects about 5 percent of people older than age 65 and 20 percent of those older than age 80. The disease destroys the brain cells concerned with memory and is associated with a reduced life expectancy. The cause of Alzheimer's disease is unknown, but several factors are thought to contribute to its development. One is a gene called apolipoprotein E4, and another is exposure to high concentrations of aluminum. Mercury in amalgam fillings does not cause Alzheimer's diesease, but it is clearly toxic to brain cells, and would not help it. Another common cause of dementia is a stroke or a series of minor strokes. This is especially common if there is high blood pressure or high blood levels of an an amino acid called homocysteine.

Keeping our memories alive

The herb gingko biloba has been shown to regulate blood flow to the brain and may boost memory and reduce confusion in older people. The same claim has been made for essential fatty acids, such as fish oil and flax oil, but the evidence is inconclusive. The Ayurvedic herb gotu kola is said to help induce mental calm and clarity, increase intelligence, and improve memory, although there is little scientific research on this. Diet is thought to be important; vitamin B_{12}, choline, and manganese may help to improve memory, and many vitamins have a positive effect on cognitive function. Naturopaths might link memory problems to food intolerances, candida of the gut, chronic fatigue syndrome, or some glandular disorders and usually suggest dietary changes and supplements. Sleeping well is also important, as is keeping the mind active, even by doing the crossword in your daily newspaper. Exercise can boost cognitive function by feeding the brain with oxygen and can help us stay alert as we age. Yoga, tai chi, and qigong are believed to increase "energy" flow—and therefore blood to the brain—and improve concentration, whereas meditation and relaxation help to calm the mind and relieve stress. Conventional drugs used to help mental function are called nootropics. The most common is paracetam; others include vinpocetine, and cetacetam.

Treating dementia

Conventional treatment for Alzheimer's disease involves drug therapy with acetylcholinesterase inhibitors, such as donepezil, rivastigmine, and galantamine. Research has shown that these drugs can delay for as much as 6–12 months the decline in thinking abilities in some people with mild to moderate disease. They are not a cure, however, and only half of people with the disease seem to benefit. They appear to block the actions of the enzyme acetylcholinesterase, which breaks down the neurotransmitter acetylcholine in the brain. The theory is that a decline in levels of this neurotransmitter is responsible for the symptoms of Alzheimer's disease. By making more acetylcholine available, the drugs can reduce symptoms.

Some studies have found the herb ginkgo biloba to be effective in delaying deterioration of thinking processes in people with Alzheimer's. Research suggests that ginkgo may be as effective as the acetylcholin esterase inhibitors used in conventional medicine, although no study has directly compared them. Some evidence shows that massage reduces anxiety and alters behavior in people with the disease, but further research is needed. Chinese medicine generally regards memory problems as a "kidney" weakness and uses herbs to boost the "kidneys". However, little research has been done on the effects of Chinese herbs or acupuncture for dementia.

eye and ear problems

As we get older, our sight and hearing can deteriorate for a number of reasons. Therefore, it is important to see a doctor as soon as possible if you have any loss of vision or persistent visual disturbance, such as flashes of light or colored haloes around lights, because they can indicate a more serious problem with your eyesight, such as macular degeneration or retinal detachment.

Strained or tired eyes

Rest is the best answer for strained or tired eyes. Make sure you take regular breaks from your computer screens to focus on a distant object for a few seconds, and make sure you are working under good lighting.

If your eyes start feeling tired at work, close them and gently press on your eyelids with your palms. Placing damp camomile or fennel tea bags or slices of cucumber over your eyes can also help. In Chinese medicine, ju hua (chrysanthemum flowers) are used to brighten and revive the eyes. Add 2 teaspoons of the dried flowers to a cup of boiled water, allow to cool, then apply to the eyes on cotton wool pads.

Sight problems

As we get older, the lenses in the eyes tend to lose elasticity, making it harder to see things clearly close up. This condition is called farsightedness, or presbyopia. It can easily be corrected with reading glasses. As you get older, it is best to have your eyes checked every 2 years for farsightedness and annually if any visual disturbance occurs. Any blurring or loss of vision should be reported to your doctor immediately.

Some complementary treatments can be used for eye problems. The herb winter cherry is reputed to be good for weak eyes, the Chinese herb ju hua is said to help improve vision, and the Ayurvedic remedy bhringaraj is supposed to rejuvenate sight, although there is little scientific evidence to support this. The Bate's method is a complementary therapy that involves special eye exercises to strengthen and reeducate the eyes. However, the evidence for its effectiveness is anecdotal.

Macular degeneration

Macular degeneration is a condition where the central part of the retina wears out because the blood vessels supplying it become narrowed. It has the effect of reducing the blood flow to the eyes, thus affecting vision. Along with old age, other causes of macular degeneration are high blood pressure, atherosclerosis, and dietary factors. Smokers are at a higher risk for this condition. Laser surgery can be of help early in the disease, but the condition is not reversible. Much can be done, however, to reduce the handicap resulting from the progressive loss of vision. Recent medical studies show that antioxidants can slow the progression of macular degeneration.

If you are older than age 40, eye exams are necessary every 2 years. Eye exams can show if corrective lenses are needed and can sometimes reveal eye disorders.

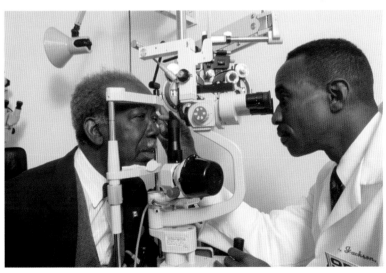

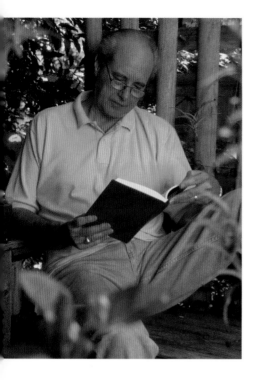

When reading, always choose a relaxing place with good light.

Glaucoma

Glaucoma is an eye disorder where pressure builds up due to reduced drainage of fluid from the eye. Untreated, it can lead to blindness. Everybody aged 40 and older should be tested for glaucoma annually, and it can be treated successfully with eyedrops, tablets, medications or surgery. Because any damage to the optic nerve that has already been caused by the buildup of pressure inside the eyeball cannot be corrected it is best to treat this condition early. The main known causes of glaucoma are aging and an inherited tendency for the disease.

Cataracts

With cataracts the lens of the eye takes on a milky appearance and becomes opaque, thereby blocking out light. Cataracts are usually due to old age, but they can also result from injury, eye disease, taking drugs such as corticosteroids, radiation, or congenital disorders. Cataracts are usually easily treated with surgery to replace the affected lens with an artificial one. Some limited evidence suggests that antioxidants like vitamins A, C, and E can help to prevent damage to the lenses by free radicals. Excessive sunlight may also cause cataracts, so it is always advisable to wear sunglasses that block both UVA and UVB from sunlight.

Presbyopia

Presbyopia is a gradual diminishing of the eye's ability to focus clearly on near objects. It is associated with aging, and develops when the lens of the eye becomes less elastic and less able to change shape to focus on objects. Presbyopia can be corrected by wearing glasses with lenses that bring light rays from objects into focus on the retina. The condition usually worsens as people get older, and it is important to have regular eye exams so that the lenses can be updated. The condition can sometimes be corrected with contact lenses. By age 60, the deterioration usually stabilizes.

Presbycusis

Presbycusis is a gradual hearing loss that is a normal consequence of aging. It usually happens after age 50, when people start to notice that they cannot hear high-pitched or quiet, soft sounds as well as before. There may also be a problem hearing conversation, especially against a background of other noises. The degree of loss can be assessed with hearing tests and, although there is no cure for the condition, hearing aids do enable people to communicate effectively.

Tinnitus

Tinnitus is a condition where there is a persistent or recurring noise in the ears, such as a ringing, buzzing, or whistling noise. About 1 in 10 people are affected. Causes include prolonged exposure to loud noise, head injuries, neck problems, ear infections, deafness, blocked ears, and Ménière's disease, which is a condition of the inner ear that causes episodes of severe vertigo, nausea, and hearing loss.

No conventional cure is available for tinnitus, but some evidence does suggest that the herb ginkgo biloba, relaxation, and hypnotherapy might help the condition. Playing background music can help to reduce awareness of the noise in the ears. In about 11 percent of cases, tinnitus clears up spontaneously.

Deafness

Loss of hearing may result from damage to the auditory nerve (nerve deafness) or to abnormalities in the external or middle ear, such as inflammation or blockage (conductive deafness). It can occur in one or both ears.

Conventional medicine treats nerve deafness with hearing aids, or in some cases, electrical implants in the cochlea, which is the receptor for hearing, located in the inner ear. Conductive deafness is aimed at removing the blockage or reducing inflammation. No conclusive evidence shows benefits from any of the complementary therapies.

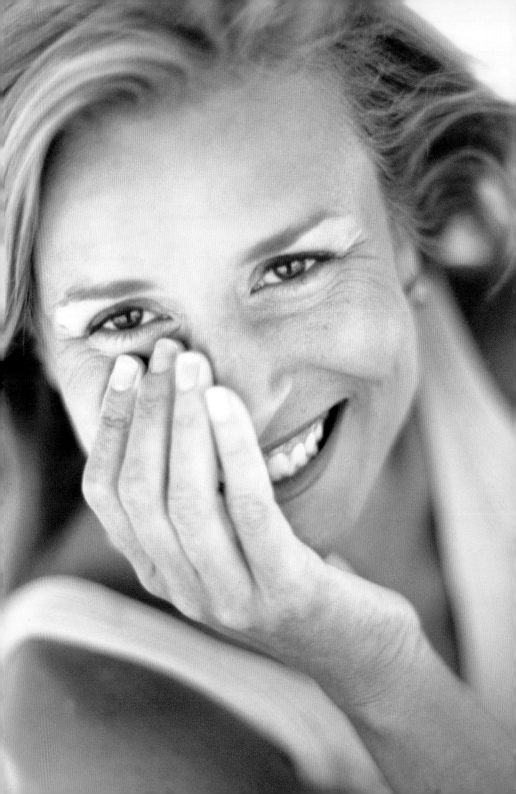

You can do various things in life to "beat the years," from changing what you eat to making sure you sleep well. In this section, we look at all the options available for taking care of your body and mind and helping you to stay young and healthy. This includes a healthy diet, exercise to keep in shape, relaxation techniques, skin and hair care, complementary therapies, and conventional medicine. Making just one change in your life can have a noticeable impact on how you feel, so don't try to change everything at once. Choose one aspect of your life—perhaps the one you think you will find the easiest to change—and see what happens.

options
for
health

taking care of yourself

Being healthy is not just about not being ill, it is about feeling full of life and energy, with your mind, body, and spirit working in harmony together. How healthy you are is partly determined by your genes but it is also influenced by what you do to yourself and the environment you live in. It is possible to achieve a high level of vitality and well-being by working out your own unique health program, through combining lifestyle and dietary measures.

The importance of emotions and the mind

Emotional and social issues can play a big part in how we grow old. One of the most important components of good health and a long life is having close, healthy ties with friends and relatives. Depression, grief, and loneliness are more common as we grow older because of retirement or because close friends and family move away or die. Social isolation has been linked to an increased risk of dying in older people who are already ill, and it has also been found to suppress the immune system, resulting in an increase in infections. Some evidence also documents that people who are depressed are more likely to develop heart disease and cancer.

Attitudes about aging and health are also important. The adage "you are only as old as you feel" has a lot of truth in it. Science and conventional medicine support many of the complementary therapies in relation to the idea that the mind and body are one unit, the mind-body or body-mind, each influencing the other. That is inseparable. So, think young!

The need to be careful

Accidents in the home, at work, and on the road are a major cause of premature death and disability. Most accidents happen in the home, and the biggest killers of older people or children are preventable accidents such as fires and drowning when left unattended in the bath. Avoiding accidents mainly comes down to common sense, but it is also about knowledge.

Living intelligently and safely can increase your chance of having a long, healthy life. Plan ahead, and give yourself time when you undertake an activity. For example, always follow the advice for safe driving. Take frequent rest breaks, always wear a seat belt when driving, don't drink and drive, wear a helmet when riding a motorbike, drive a big car, and keep well within the allocated speed limit.

Look at the following questions in the How healthy are you? box. Do you answer "yes" to any of them? If you did, you might consider trying to change these things in your life to bring some health benefits.

HOW HEALTHY ARE YOU?

- *Do you smoke tobacco or take other recreational drugs?*
- *Are you overweight for your height? Your body mass index (BMI) is your weight in kilograms divided by the square of your height in meters. It is an estimate of your total body fat. The standard is that people with a BMI between 25 and 29.9 kilograms per meter squared (kg/m^2) are overweight, those with a BMI of 30–39.9 kg/m^2 are obese, and those with a BMI of 40 kg/m^2 or more are severely obese.*
- *Is your pulse more than 85–90 beats per minute if you are a man, or more than 95–100 beats per minute if you are a woman?*
- *Do you eat a lot of sugary, fatty, fried, or processed foods?*
- *Do you drink more than one drink a day (women) or two drinks a day (men)—one drink is 12 oz of beer, a glass of wine, or $1^1/_2$ oz of spirits?*
- *Do you have high blood pressure, cholesterol, or glucose levels?*
- *Are you a couch potato, rarely exercising?*
- *Are you stressed out, finding it hard to relax and unwind?*
- *Do you find it hard to sleep and wake up feeling tired or unrested?*
- *Are you lonely, with few close friends or family?*

nutrition and healthy eating

Today, healthy eating messages can be seen everywhere and are aimed at everyone. However, most people can make improvements with a few simple changes to their diet.

Research has shown that certain diets can increase your risk of getting heart disease, having a stroke, or developing certain cancers. If you have an illness, what you eat can also affect whether you get better or how bad the symptoms are. For many people, one of the biggest benefits of a healthy diet is weight loss. Obesity is one of the biggest health problems in the industrialized world because it increases your risk of getting heart disease, diabetes, certain cancers, and arthritis.

What is a healthy diet?

A healthy diet should include the right proportion and type of carbohydrates, proteins, fats, vitamins, and minerals (see p.58) to give the body energy and all the nutrients it needs for growth and repair. To develop a healthy diet, keep these simple rules in mind:

• Eat at least five portions of fruit and vegetables a day (except potatoes because they are high in carbohydrates). This isn't as hard as it sounds. For example, if you have a glass of fruit juice with your breakfast, a side salad and a piece of fruit with your lunch, and two vegetables with your evening meal, you've done it.

• Eat less fat. Fat should make up only about 30 percent of daily calories, and only 10 percent should come from saturated fats. Trans fats should not be in our diets at all.

• Eat more fiber, and make sure that about 50 percent of your calories come from complex carbohydrates, found in whole grains and vegetables, and starchy foods like pasta, bread, rice, potatoes, dried beans and legumes, and cereals. You will probably find that as you increase the amount of these foods, you will eat less fatty ones.

- Eat less sugar. It gives you energy but no other nutrients. One of the best ways to lose weight is to reduce the amount of sugary foods you eat.
- Decrease your intake of sodium because a high-sodium diet can lead to high blood pressure. Don't add salt to food during cooking or at the table, and avoid manufactured foods high in salt, such as canned foods, chips and other snacks.
- Get your protein from fish, poultry, legumes, cereal, and low-fat dairy products rather than red meat. Only 15 percent of your daily calories need come from protein.
- Avoid processed and "junk" foods, because these are more likely to contain additives like preservatives, colorings, and flavorings, which may increase your risk of cancer. Be aware that "natural" additives are not necessarily more healthy.

What about unsaturated fats?

Although a healthy diet involves minimizing the total amount of fat you consume, some oil in the diet is essential. Unsaturated fat—such as that found in sunflower or olive oil, nuts, seeds, and oily fish—is best. The two types of unsaturated fats are monosaturated, such as found in olive oil, and polyunsaturated, which includes omega-6 oils found in plant oils like sunflower or soybean oils. These fats can actually help to lower cholesterol levels, and because the omega-3 oils in flax seed oil and fatty fish help to make the blood less sticky and less likely to clot, they protect against heart attack and stroke. These are known as essential fatty acids. A healthy diet should include at least one to two portions of oily fish (such as mackerel, sardines, or herring) every week. Saturated animal fats should be avoided because they increase the risk of heart and circulatory diseases (see p.22). If you do eat meat, make sure it's lean.

Saturated fats are solid at room temperature, and unsaturated fats are liquid. To harden unsaturated fats to make margarines and baked goods, manufacturers hydrogenate them. This process converts the unsaturated fats into either saturated fats or into transaturated fats and strips the unsaturated fats of their health benefits.

What about fiber?

Fiber, which is found in plant foods, is not broken down in the gut but passes through it without being absorbed. It can help to soften and increase the bulk of stools, thus preventing constipation. Two types of fiber exist. Insoluble fiber is found in rice, whole grains, dried fruit, and nuts, and it shortens the time it takes for food to pass through the intestines, which may help to prevent the buildup of cancer-causing substances and so reduce the risk of colon cancer. Soluble fiber is found in fruit and vegetables, dried beans and legumes, and oat bran. It appears to reduce the amount of cholesterol absorbed into the body from food and so helps to reduce the risk of heart disease. Soluble fiber also slows glucose absorption into the bloodstream and thus can help to control blood glucose levels (see p.29).

What about water?

A healthy diet also includes drinking at least eight 8-ounce (237-milliliter) glasses of water a day to prevent the skin from becoming dull and dry and to flush out toxins from the body. Water gives bulk to soluble fiber in the large intestine, helping to prevent constipation and keeping the bowels healthy. The more fiber you eat, the more important it is to drink lots of water. Some people believe that pure distilled water is best because it actively detoxifies the body and that distilling water can rid it of fluorides, pesticides, chlorine, and heavy metals; however, little scientific evidence supports this theory.

Protecting against disease

Research suggests that about 35–60 percent of all cancer deaths are linked to diet. Certain diets may increase the risk of cancer, whereas others may protect against it. Diets high in fat, particularly saturated fats, seem to increase the risk of breast, colon, and prostate cancers. Charring food during grilling or barbecuing produces potential cancer-inducing substances (such as nitrosamines).

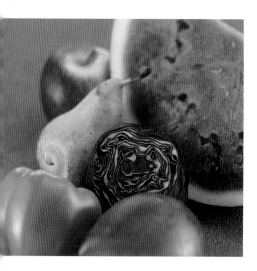

Cancers of the breast, uterus, and gallbladder are also more common in people who are overweight. Diets rich in fruits and vegetables seem to protect against some cancers. Green leafy vegetables and red and orange fruit and vegetables are

Many fruits and vegetables give protection against some cancers.

good sources of antioxidants (see p.58), which "mop up" harmful substances in the body. Red peppers and tomatoes may reduce the risk of cervical and prostate cancers. Broccoli and other brassicas may protect against breast, prostate and uterine cancers, and garlic and onions may help prevent digestive tract and bladder cancers. Whole-grain cereals, sunflower seeds, oysters, and other shellfish are also good sources of antioxidants and may help to protect against cancer.

Although a diet low in saturated fats is healthy, dairy products like milk and cheese are a good source of calcium, which protects against osteoporosis. Low-fat and nonfat dairy products are good choices because they are low in fat but don't have significantly reduced mineral levels.

Losing weight and using nutrition therapy

The principles of healthy eating are the same for people who want to lose weight as for those who want to stay healthy. Although healthy eating may only change your size and shape slowly, it retrains your taste buds and your body, which may be a permanent effect. Many crash dieters, on the other hand, end up going back to old eating habits and regaining all the weight they have lost. Nutrition therapy is the science of treating disease and restoring health by using specific dietary factors and supplements, and cutting out toxins and allergens. See naturopathy (see p.130).

Understanding food sensitivities

The two types of food sensitivity are allergies and intolerance. Food allergies are relatively rare but can be life-threatening, and they usually last a lifetime. If you are allergic to a food, your immune system reacts as if it is a harmful substance. The signs and symptoms of a food allergy can range from hives (nettle rash), vomiting, and diarrhea to the symptoms of IBS, migraine or asthma, and anaphylactic shock, when the chest tightens and breathing becomes difficult; the lips, mouth, and tongue swell; and collapse, or even death, can result. Food intolerance can disappear if the food causing the intolerance is cut out of the diet for a few months. These problems require the expertise of specialist physicians. Such intolerance can cause a blocked nose, headaches, tiredness, emotional problems, joint or muscle pain, stomach upsets with bloating, cramping pains, nausea and indigestion, skin problems, and water retention. Elimination diets are not recommended unless you are allergic, and they require medical supervision.

vitamins and minerals

If we eat a healthy and well-balanced diet, we should have no need for vitamin or mineral supplements. Doctors and scientists at the World Health Organization have set a recommended daily allowance (RDA) for many vitamins and minerals. However, these allowances are set at levels that prevent diseases, such as scurvy due to lack of vitamin C and rickets due to lack of vitamin D, rather than at levels that maintain optimum health.

Vital nutrients

Research has suggested that mass production of food in the industrialized, polluted world destroys some nutrients, and some experts believe that we need to take increased amounts of certain supplements to keep healthy. Our need for supplements depends on age, environment, whether we are ill or pregnant, and even genetics. In the United States, for instance, only a third of the population gets all the RDAs through diet. Experts agree that we should try to get the vitamins and minerals we need from our diet but acknowledge that most of us do not.

Antioxidants

The main antioxidants are the ACE vitamins—vitamin A (as beta carotene), C, and E—and the minerals copper, manganese, selenium, and zinc. Research has suggested that antioxidants can protect against premature aging, cancer, and heart disease and that they may be beneficial for arthritis and asthma. Antioxidants find and "mop up" free radicals in the body. Free radicals are molecules our bodies create as defense against bacteria, but can also be increased in response to cigarette smoke, chemicals, and industrial pollution. Although alive for just a few seconds, they can damage DNA (genetic material) in cells and affect cholesterol so that it is more likely to stick to artery walls. These actions can make us more susceptible to cancer and to heart and circulatory disorders. Although our bodies do make some antioxidants, we probably could all do with more.

Supplements and growing older

As we get older, we need fewer calories and so need less food. However, we still need as many vitamins and minerals from our diet as we always have. In addition, the absorption of nutrients (such as zinc, pyridoxine, and vitamin D) is often reduced as we get older, and this can lessen our feelings of well-being and weaken the body's immune system. As we age, the following supplements can help:

Vitamin A can help to remove age spots.

Thiamine, riboflavin, and **pyridoxine** may help to prevent premature aging.

Vitamin B₁₂, choline, and **manganese** can help to improve memory.

Biotin, choline, and **folic acid** may help to stop hair from turning gray

Biotin and **inositol** can help prevent baldness.

Vitamin C can stop skin wrinkling, bruising, and broken veins under the skin.

Vitamin D and **calcium** help to prevent osteoporosis.

Vitamins A, C, and **E, copper, manganese, selenium,** and **zinc** can help keep you look younger through their antioxidant action.

Iodine and **zinc** can improve mental alertness.

Co-enzyme Q10 is an important supplement for energy production. It is found in all of the body's tissues and organs. Research suggests that we may become deficient in co-enzyme Q10 as we get older, leading to reduced energy levels.

Chondroitin and **glucosamine** may be helpful for arthritic problems (see p.34).

Omega-3 and **omega-6 oils,** also known as essential fatty acids (EFAs), may be helpful for arthritic problems (see p.34) and may help prevent heart and circulatory disease (see p.22).

DMSO (dimethyl sulphoxide) and **MSM (methyl sulphonyl methane)** may be helpful for arthritic problems. Many people have used DMSO to treat arthritis, because it penetrates through the skin and has anti-inflammatory effects. About 15 percent of absorbed DMSO is converted to MSM, which some clinicians and researchers believe is responsible for the therapeutic effects. At least some of its effect is thought to come from its rich sulfur content. MSM is present in many foods and is widely available as a supplement. Its recommended uses include the treatment of arthritis and soft-tissue injuries. It is taken orally, and clinicians suggest dosages starting at 500 mg twice a day with meals, building up to 2–8 g daily.

Vitamins

Vitamins are organic substances that are only found in living things. They are essential in small amounts for human growth and the maintenance of good health. However, we cannot make them ourselves and must get them from what we eat. Pregnant women should consult their health care professional about which supplements they need to take and which ones they should avoid.

Vitamin A (beta carotene) is needed for good night vision, healthy skin, and normal growth. It is also an antioxidant. Good sources are liver, oily fish, green leafy vegetables, carrots, tomatoes, apricots, eggs, butter, cheese, and milk.

Thiamine (B_1) turns fat, sugar, and protein into energy and helps maintain brain function. Good sources are potatoes, whole grains, brown rice, vegetables, milk, dried beans and legumes, nuts, fish, and meat.

Riboflavin (B_2) turns fat, sugar, and protein into energy and is needed for healthy skin, hair, nails, and eyes. Good sources are almonds, wild rice, soybeans, lentils, broccoli, whole-grain bread, mackerel, milk, eggs, yogurt, liver, and other meat.

Niacin (B_3) is needed for energy production, helps to control blood glucose and cholesterol levels, and is important for the nervous system. Good sources are oily fish, whole wheat, asparagus, almonds, brown rice, dairy products, liver, and other meat.

Pantothenic acid (B_5) is involved in energy production and helps maintain the nervous and immune systems and the skin. Good sources include whole wheat, alfalfa sprouts, peas, lentils, nuts, eggs, mushrooms, brown rice, milk, liver, and kidneys.

Pyridoxine (B_6) helps with the digestion of protein and is important in maintaining hormone balance, the immune system, and brain function. Good sources are brown rice, whole grains, cauliflower, fish, soybeans, sweet potatoes, sunflower seeds, oranges, bananas, eggs, and meat.

Cobalamin (B_{12}) is needed to maintain healthy red blood cells and to protect nerves. Good sources are fish, shellfish, meat, milk, cheese, and eggs.

Biotin is needed to produce energy from fat and to help maintain the glands

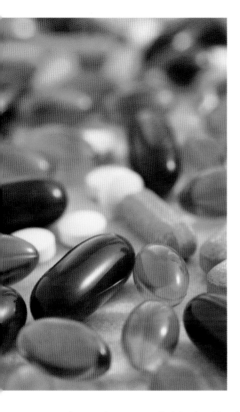

that produce sex hormones. Good sources are liver, lentils, pork, kidneys, eggs, nuts, cauliflower, brown rice, and whole grains.

Choline helps with the breakdown of fats. Good sources are eggs, cauliflower, cucumber, and peanuts.

Inositol helps to transport fat from the liver. Good sources are soy products, eggs, citrus fruits, whole grains, and nuts.

Folic acid is needed for healthy blood cells and during pregnancy to prevent birth defects such as spina bifida. It is also thought to enhance memory. Good sources are leafy green vegetables, potatoes, dried beans and legumes, nuts, citrus fruits, and liver.

Vitamin C (ascorbic acid) helps the body to absorb iron and aids the healing of wounds. It is needed for healthy skin, gums, teeth, and bones and is also an antioxidant. Good sources are citrus fruits, black currants, strawberries, kiwi fruit, mango, leafy green vegetables, potatoes, and tomatoes.

Vitamin D helps the body absorb calcium to keep teeth and bones healthy. Good sources are sunlight, margarine, oily fish, eggs, butter, and brown rice.

Vitamin E is an antioxidant that protects body tissue against free radicals. Good sources are nuts, seeds, vegetables oils, eggs, butter, avocados, asparagus, olives, spinach, blackberries, salmon, and tuna.

Vitamin K regulates blood-clotting factors, which includes both excessive bleeding and clotting. Good sources are leafy green vegetables, especially kale, broccoli, green cabbage, brussels sprouts, and watercress; egg yolk; cod-liver oil; and soybean oil.

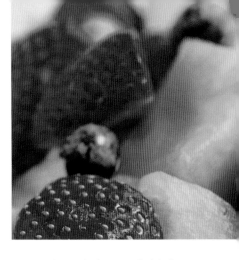

Soft fruits are a good source of vitamin C.

Minerals and trace elements

Minerals are found in soil and are absorbed by plants and anything that eats those plants. Like vitamins, minerals are essential for health. Water is not a significant source of minerals. The two types of minerals are those we need in amounts of more than 100 mg a day, which are called bulk minerals, and those we need in small amounts, which are known as trace elements.

Minerals

Calcium is essential for more than 300 enzyme reactions in the body and is necessary to maintain healthy bones and teeth, normal transmission of nerve impulses, clotting blood, and maintainenance of normal heart function. Good sources are dairy products, tofu, sardines, watercress, parsley, dried figs, almonds, dried apricots, cabbage, oatmeal, and sesame seeds.

Magnesium maintains strong bones and teeth, regulates the heartbeat, calms the nervous system, and regulates thyroid function. Good sources are spinach, figs, nuts, dried beans and legumes, wheat germ, sardines, sweet corn, bananas, and milk.

Phosphorus, which is present in every cell, is involved in virtually every process that takes place in the body. It is also needed for strong teeth and bones. Good sources are fish, meat, whole grains, eggs, nuts, and seeds.

Potassium works with sodium to regulate the body's water balance and to regulate the heartbeat. It is also needed for nerve and muscle function. Good sources are citrus fruits, watercress, leafy green vegetables, bananas, melons, and potatoes.

Sodium works with potassium. We obtain most of our sodium from salt. The average person consumes excessive amounts of salt in their diet.

Trace elements

Chromium maintains balanced blood glucose levels, controls cravings and hunger. Good sources are wheat germ, meat, shellfish, eggs, apples, and parsnips.

Chloride works with sodium and potassium and also helps the liver detoxify the body. Good sources are table salt, kelp, and olives.

Copper helps make red blood cells. Good sources are dried beans and legumes, peas, whole wheat, prunes, liver, and most seafood.

Iodine is mainly involved in the proper functioning of the thyroid gland. Good sources are kelp, vegetables grown in iodine-rich soil, onions, and seafood.

Iron is needed for healthy red blood cells to prevent anemia. Good sources are red meat, liver, seafood, fish, cereals, beans, dried fruit, nuts, and bread. Iron supplements should be avoided by men and postmenopausal women.

Manganese helps balance blood glucose levels and is important for good metabolism, bone growth, and healthy thyroid function. Good sources are fruit, almonds, whole grains, brussels sprouts, carrots, and eggs.

Selenium is an antioxidant, and is important in the prevention of cancer. Good sources are meat, Brazil nuts, oily fish, bread, and rice.

Sulfur is essential for healthy hair, skin, and nails and proper brain and liver function. Good sources are beef, dried beans and legumes, fish, eggs, and cabbage.

Zinc is needed for many hormones, including insulin, to function correctly. It helps keep blood glucose levels balanced, and it is also necessary for fertility, helping cells to divide and grow. It is vital for normal immune function. Good sources are rye, oats, almonds, peas, milk, fish, seafood, meat, and turkey.

Can vitamins and minerals be dangerous?

Anything taken to excess is toxic; however the fat soluble vitamins A, D, E, and K are fat-soluble and can be stored in excessive amounts of some of them, particularly vitamin A, which is known to cause toxicity. In addition, taking large doses of other supplements can have adverse effects. For example, large doses of vitamin C can cause diarrhea, too much niacin (B_3) or pyridoxine (B_6) can cause nerve and liver damage, and more than 15 mg of folic acid can cause digestive upsets and sleep problems. In the case of minerals, more than 1,000 mg of magnesium a day can cause low blood pressure, diarrhea, and flushing. High doses of potassium and selenium are toxic. However, toxic reactions from vitamin and mineral supplements are rare, and if you take a high-quality multivitamin and follow the guidelines on the label, you should not encounter any problems.

keeping in shape

Regular exercise helps keep us fit and healthy looking, but exercise isn't just about keeping trim. It improves our energy and well-being and can increase our life expectancy. It improves the function of the heart and lungs, keeps joints mobile and improves posture, strengthens our muscles to give us more stamina, and increases blood circulation so that our skin looks healthier. Exercise can boost mental capacity by feeding the brain with oxygen, helping us to stay alert as we get older. However, if you stop exercising, the benefits you have gained can be lost within weeks.

The commitment to exercise

There is little point in putting effort into getting fit if you fail to keep it up, so always choose activities that you enjoy and can fit easily into your lifestyle. Try to incorporate exercise into your everyday life—walk instead of getting the bus or take the stairs rather than the elevator. Variety will help stop you getting bored. It is also a good idea to have indoor and outdoor activity options so that a rainy day doesn't give you the excuse not to exercise. Remember, you're never to old to start exercising.

Exercise and disease prevention

Research has shown that regular exercise reduces the risk of diabetes, lowers high blood pressure and cholesterol levels, facilitates weight loss, and improves the function of the heart, all of which helps to prevent heart disease and strokes (see p.22). Studies have also found that exercise keeps joints mobile, helping to prevent arthritis and rheumatism (see p.34) , and strengthens muscles and bones, reducing the risk of falls, fractures, and osteoporosis (see p.36). Evidence also shows that regular exercise can reduce the risk of colon cancer and, possibly, breast and prostate cancers too.

Exercise and well-being

Regular exercise can help to reduce stress and anxiety and improve sleep. Research has shown that it can be as effective as psychotherapy or antidepressants for mild depression. When we exercise, the body's natural opiates, or endorphins, are released and lift our mood. Alpha brain waves associated with relaxation (see p.82) become more dominant. Improved body awareness and body shape that comes from regular exercise can give us a sense of well-being.

What is physical fitness?

To keep in shape, we need to have cardiovascular fitness, muscular endurance, and strength and flexibility, and to get these benefits, we must exercise regularly. Therefore, we need 30 minutes of aerobic exercise five times a week to improve our health. Vigorous aerobic exercise—such as fast walking, jogging, or cycling—improves cardiovascular fitness. Aerobic means "with oxygen." During aerobic exercise, the large muscles in the arms, legs, and back expand and contract at a steady pace. To keep going, the muscles need more oxygen. You start breathing faster and more deeply to take more oxygen into your blood, and your heart beats faster to pump the extra oxygen around your body more rapidly. This exercises your heart and lungs and they become more efficient. Muscular endurance is developed by exercising large muscle groups repeatedly, such as in circuit training or swimming. Brief bursts of intensive activity (anaerobic exercise), such as weight lifting, increases muscle strength. Stretching muscles improves flexibility, for example, with yoga (see p.114) or warm-up exercises.

Is it aerobic or not?

To calculate whether the exercise you are doing is aerobic or not, you can estimate your optimum heart rate during exercise. It should be 60–80 percent of your maximum heart rate, or roughly 220 minus your age. As you become fitter, you will need to increase the intensity of exercise to maintain your optimum heart rate. To work out your heart rate, place two fingers on the pulse found on the thumb side of your inner wrist or on the side of your neck. Count the beats for 60 seconds. A simpler way to tell if you are exercising aerobically is to exercise until you are slightly out of breath and your heart beats a bit faster than normal, but you still have enough breath to talk.

Which activity should I choose?

One of the simplest ways of increasing the amount of exercise you do is to walk briskly instead of driving. This has many benefits: It can save you money, it is doing what the human body is well designed to do, and it integrates exercise into your daily life. Cycling also has many of the benefits of walking, and it can get you around quicker. Everyday activities done with vigor can improve fitness, such as washing the car, cleaning windows, gardening, painting and decorating, or cleaning in the home.

Aerobic exercises

You can do many activities on your own to increase your amount of aerobic exercise. Skipping, jogging, running, swimming, and skating are good examples. However, people often realize that they're unlikely to keep going without support from other people. If you think this might be true for you, try exercising with a friend or join an exercise class or health club. There are lots of classes that improve aerobic fitness, such as step classes, aerobics, and dancing (from salsa and tango to ballet and jazz). Racket sports (like badminton, squash, and tennis) and team games (like football, volleyball, and hockey) can also help you keep fit. However, don't overdo things in an attempt to win if you are just beginning to get fit.

Exercises that improve muscle tone

It is also important to improve the condition of your muscles. Making them stronger and more supple and improving their endurance can help to protect them and the bones against injury. All the aerobic exercises already mentioned can help strengthen muscles and give you more stamina. Simple stretching exercises and such practices as yoga (see p.114), Pilates, or tai chi help to stretch muscles and increase their strength. Weight lifting can strengthen specific muscles.

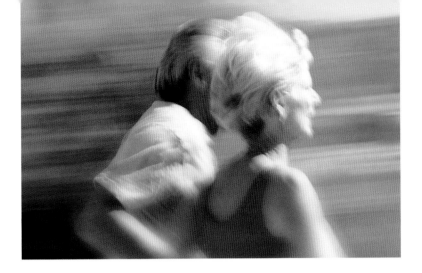

Regular exercise can improve your fitness. It reduces the risk of getting many diseases, as well as keeping joints mobile and strengthening the bones.

How much exercise should I do?

If you are already fit and exercise regularly, you can probably start exercising aerobically for 30 minutes, five times a week; however, if you are unfit or older, you should begin with small amounts and gradually build up to avoid injury. If you feel pain when you're exercising, you have overdone things and should stop. Although muscles may feel sore after exercising, especially if you haven't been active for a while, it is best to consult your doctor about any pain that fails to go away.

When should I consult my doctor?

See your doctor *before* you start exercising if you:

- have high blood pressure or high cholesterol levels.
- suffer from heart disease.
- have a respiratory disorder like asthma.
- suffer with back trouble.
- have arthritis or other joint problems.
- are diabetic.
- are recovering from an illness or operation.
- are pregnant.
- are very overweight.
- are a heavy smoker.

simple

exercises

to do at home

Warm up for 5–15 minutes before embarking on any
physically demanding activity. A good routine should
warm up your whole body and get you slightly sweating,
and it should increase blood flow through your tissues,
making them more elastic and ready for action. Include
movements in your warm-up routine that you will be doing
during your main physical activity. For example, if you are
going to play golf, practice your swing with an imaginary
golf club and ball. Stretching exercises can be carried
out at anytime, to improve your flexibility. The following
pages contain basic warm-ups, stretches, and advice
for how to conduct an exercise program.

Limbering up

Step 1—upper limbs Circle your shoulders backward and forward. Stretch your
arms out and rotate at your shoulders, followed by elbows and then wrists, first in
one direction, then in the other. Stretch your arms out in front of you. Finally, wiggle
your fingers, and give your hands a good shake.

Step 2—lower limbs Straighten one leg out, lifting it a little way off the floor
and gently swing it backward and forward, and round in small circles. Wiggle your
toes, and circle the foot in one direction and then the other. Repeat with the other
foot. Finally, give your legs a gentle shake.

Step 3—the neck Let your head hang loosely forward toward your chest. Slowly rotate it, first to one side, then to the other in a half circle. Repeat this about three times. Look down at all times. Do not twist your neck or take your head backward, because this can damage your spine.

Step 4—the spine Stand up straight with your feet about 2 feet (61 centimeters) apart and pointing forward. Keeping your knees soft and slightly bent, swing your arms from side to side, twisting your trunk but keeping the area below your hips facing forward. Twist in this way 5–10 times.

Stretching out

The calf muscles In a standing position, step forward about 3 feet (91.5 centimeters) with your right leg, and bend its knee until you can feel a stretch on the calf of your left (back) leg. Both your feet should be flat on the floor and your left (back) leg should be straight. Lean forward, keeping your stomach and back straight, and rest your hands on your right (front) knee. Hold for a count of 10 and then repeat with the other leg in front.

The hamstrings In a standing position, step forward about 2 feet (61 centimeters) with your right leg, and then shift your weight on to your left (back) leg. Straighten your right (front) leg, then bend your left (back). Rest your hands on your right (front) leg for support. Both your feet should be flat on the floor. You should feel a stretch up the back of your right (front) leg. Hold for a count of 10, and repeat with the other leg.

The quadriceps Stand on your left leg and bend the right knee up so that its heel comes close to your right buttock. You should feel a stretch in your right front thigh. Grasp the ankle with your right hand, and hold for a count of 10. Repeat with the left leg. If you find balancing difficult, you can support yourself by placing your free hand against a wall.

The shoulders Stand with your feet about 2 feet (61 centimeters) apart. Bend your right arm across your chest, resting its wrist on the left shoulder. Gently push your upper right arm with the left hand under the elbow of the right arm. This stretches out the back of your shoulders. Hold for a count of 5. Repeat about five times on each arm. Still standing with your feet apart, clasp your hands behind your back, and then raise your arms up as high as you can, keeping your back straight. This stretches out the front of your shoulders. Hold for a count of 10. Repeat twice.

Getting your heart working

March up and down or gently jog on the spot for a few minutes, lifting your knees up as fast as you can. This exercise can be done at home or even at work. Alternatively, walk up and down the stairs a few times. This gets your heart pumping a little faster, your lungs working harder, and your blood circulating better, in preparation for the physical activity to come.

Cooling down

How you end an exercise session is just as important as how you begin it. When muscles have been active, they need to cool down gradually. Cooling down also brings the heart rate back to normal slowly, and this prevents pooling of blood in the legs. Cooling down gradually also helps to keep extra blood flowing through the muscles so that it can carry away waste products of exercise such as lactic acid. If this is left in the muscles, it can make them stiff or sore. A good way to cool down

Tai chi is a Chinese movement therapy consisting of sequences of slow movements and breathing techniques. It is said to improve the flow of qi (see acupuncture, p.100), or energy, around the body and enhance health and fitness. It can promote relaxation and help posture, flexibility, and balance.

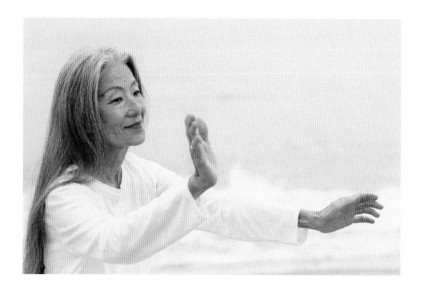

is by reducing the intensity of the activity you have been doing (be it running, cycling, or swimming) before slowing down to a stop. Walking at a slow pace for 5 minutes until your breathing slows down to normal is also recommended, perhaps gently shaking your legs and arms every now and then as you walk. At the end of your cool down, repeat some of the stretching exercises that you did in your warm up, but try to hold them a little longer.

Some strengthening exercises

Sit-ups Sit-ups strengthen stomach and back muscles. Lie on your back with your legs bent up, but keep your feet flat on the floor about hip-width apart. Contract your stomach muscles so that the lower back is flat on the floor. Either clasp your hands lightly behind your head or stretch your arms out toward your knees. Keeping your chin in and stomach muscles pulled in, curl your body up from the floor. Breathe out as you curl up, and breathe in as you go back to the floor. Repeat up to 30 times. Stop if you feel any strain in your neck.

Back strengthener Strengthen your back muscles by lying face down on the floor with your hands behind your head, then while keeping your hips on the floor, lift your head and upper body up. Hold for a count of 5, and repeat at least three times.

Exercise tips

• Always warm up for 5–15 minutes before starting aerobic exercise. This helps to stretch muscles and reduce the risk of injury.

• Cool down after exercise with slower movements and stretching exercises. This helps to prevent muscle cramps and stiffness.

• Build up gradually, especially if you have not exercised for a while. Never force yourself if the exercise seems difficult.

• Don't give yourself unrealistic goals that will reduce your motivation.

• Drink plenty of fluids during and after exercise, even if you don't feel thirsty. This replaces any fluids lost through sweating.

• Stop if you feel any pain.

• Don't do vigorous exercise if you have a cold or feel unwell.

sports

With so many different sports to choose from, it is best to think about what you like when selecting one that is perfect for you. Most important, consider what the sport will do for you in terms of your stamina, strength, and suppleness. For example, tennis is an aerobic exercise which, if played regularly, strengthens muscles, improves bone strength and density, and helps with joint mobility.

Sports

Bowls, darts, fishing, and pool are all light, nonaerobic activities and therefore don't have much effect on stamina, suppleness, or strength.

Circuit training is a moderate activity if you don't get out of breath or sweaty but a vigorous one if you do. It can improve stamina, suppleness, and strength, but it depends on the quality and routine of the class.

Cycling is a moderate activity if you don't get out of breath or sweaty but a vigorous one if you do. It is particularly good for building stamina, and it has some effect on strength but little effect on suppleness. It is always advisable to wear a helmet when cycling.

Football is a moderate activity if you don't get out of breath or sweaty but a vigorous one if you do. It has some effect on stamina, suppleness, and strength.

Golf is a light activity if you don't get out of breath or sweaty but a moderate activity if you do. It has little effect on stamina but some effect on suppleness and strength. It is probably a good idea to have a few lessons when you begin.

Long-distance walking (2 or more miles) at an average or slow pace is a light activity; at a brisk or fast pace, a moderate activity. Walking and rambling have some effect on stamina. Hill walking is vigorous and has some effect on strength.

Rowing is a good exercise for building stamina and has some effect on strength. However, it has little effect on suppleness and can aggravate a bad back.

Running is a moderate activity if you don't get out of breath or sweaty but a vigorous one if you do. It is good for building stamina but has little effect on suppleness and strength. It is important to wear proper, well-fitting running shoes and to run on grass rather than on pavement or road, if possible.

Social dancing is a light activity if you don't get out of breath or sweaty but a moderate activity if you do. Ballroom dancing has some effect on suppleness but little effect on stamina and strength. Disco dancing has some effect on stamina.

Squash, badminton, and **tennis** are moderate activities if you don't get out of breath or sweaty but vigorous ones if you do. These sports all have some effect at building stamina, suppleness, and strength, particularly squash. Table tennis is a light activity if you don't get out of breath or sweaty but a moderate activity if you do.

Swimming is a moderate activity if you don't get out of breath or sweaty but a vigorous one if you do. Hard swimming is the best all-around exercise, as it can improve stamina, suppleness, and strength.

Weight training can improve strength, but it has little effect on stamina and suppleness. It is important that you are properly supervised if you weight train.

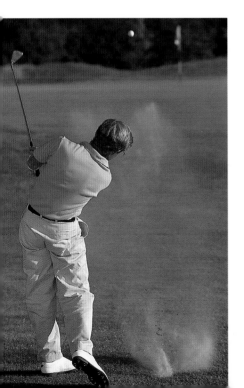

Injuries

Sports injury is common as sport grows more popular. Rugby, football, and hockey are the most injury-prone, followed by cricket and the martial arts. Racket sports are next, then horse riding, running, weight training, and swimming. Common injuries include:

- tenderness and swelling
- bruising
- cuts and abrasions
- blisters
- sprains and strains
- dislocations and fractures.

Golf is a light or moderate activity that can improve suppleness and strength.

posture

Most of us pick up bad postural habits during our lives, many of which begin in childhood. We may slouch when we're sitting down, bend at our waists rather than at the knees when we pick something up off the floor, or stare at the floor as we walk. All of these bad habits can lead to problems such as back pain, neck pain, headaches, and joint conditions such as arthritis. Bad posture can also prevent us from breathing correctly, which can lead to poor health, tiredness, and stress.

Good posture gives us a sense of freedom, ease of movement, increased well-being, and more energy. It is never too late to improve your posture. There are several methods you can try—such as the Alexander technique, Feldenkrais method, Hellerwork, Rolfing (see p.76), and yoga (see p.114)—to improve your posture. If you have a problem like lower back pain due to poor posture, treatments such as chiropractic manipulation and osteopathy (see p.108) can also be helpful.

The Alexander technique

The Alexander technique teaches you how to hold yourself more efficiently and to develop a posture that is beneficial to your health, regardless of whether you are sitting, standing, walking, or even talking. These actions use many different muscles, and the Alexander technique teaches body awareness so that you can move and hold these muscles in the most efficient way.

The technique was developed by the actor Frederick Alexander, after he found that the way he stood affected his breathing and his voice. By carefully observing himself in a full-length mirror and experimenting with his posture, he discovered that good posture is the most efficient use of the skeleton to keep the body erect and give it freedom of movement. In short, it depends on a balanced relationship between the head, neck, and spine, and is a way of standing, sitting, or moving that does not put excessive strain on the muscles or joints anywhere in the body.

How can it help? As well as improving your posture and making you aware of your body, the Alexander technique is also restful and calming. It can help you regain psychological and physical poise. By releasing tension and improving breathing and the circulation of blood and lymph, the technique can help relieve ailments such as back pain, joint problems, headaches, breathing problems, stress, and anxiety.

Learning the technique The Alexander technique is an educational process for learning how to change your postural habits, and it is best learned through the guidance of a qualified teacher.

The objective is to maintain balance through the poise of the head and total lengthening of the spine at rest and while moving. In the first lesson, the teacher will observe you, noting how you move, sit, and stand. By making adjustments to your body at rest and while you are doing everyday activities, such as standing up from a chair, the teacher helps you increase your awareness of how you move and puts you in touch with your body.

A good posture comes from within and it cannot be forced on your body. In subsequent lessons, which will be tailored to suit your needs, you will probably be taught ways of moving, bending, and reaching, combined with some relaxation to help you let go of excess tension. The teacher may also help you with specific movements that relate to your work or lifestyle, such as how to sit while playing a musical instrument or how to write without causing excess tension, work at a computer, pick up heavy items, or carry heavy bags.

Feldenkrais method

The aim of the Feldenkrais method is to restore full efficiency and functioning of the body. Developed by Moshe Feldenkrais, this method is a synthesis of some aspects of the Alexander technique and some concepts from Oriental martial arts such as judo.

The method consists of a series of well thought out and sophisticated exercises that increase body awareness in movement. As well as improving posture and general well-being, the Feldenkrais method can help with a range of muscle, joint, or nerve problems, and it can also improve breathing. In common with the

Alexander technique, it is best learned from a qualified teacher, who may also use gentle manipulation during the lessons, particularly if you have neurological conditions such as multiple sclerosis.

Hellerwork

Hellerwork combines deep massage and manipulation with reeducation about the way the body moves; it also involves exploration of emotional issues. The therapy was developed by Joseph Heller, who worked with Dr. Ida Rolf (see below) and shared her ideas concerning body alignment and ways of releasing muscle tension. However, Heller also emphasized the importance of the psychological and

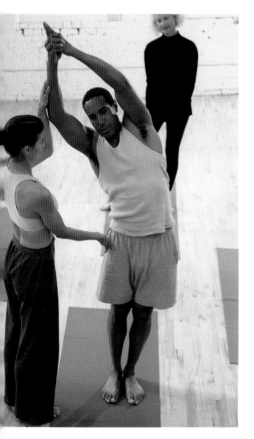

emotional aspects of health and illness, believing that we store emotional traumas in our bodies, which can eventually lead to rigidity and tension. During a session, the teacher and patient explore the emotions triggered when this tension is released. Rolfing is mainly used to improve posture and treat muscle pain, breathing problems, stress, and sports injuries. Hellerwork is inappropriate for those suffering from cancer, rheumatoid arthritis, or other inflammatory conditions.

Rolfing

Rolfing, named after its inventor Dr. Ida Rolf, is also known as structural integration. It consists of physical manipulation and postural release, which is aimed at realigning the body and releasing muscle tension. During a session, the teacher will

Therapies such as Hellerwork and Rolfing help to correct poor posture.

Our spines should not be poker straight. Instead, a spine is made up of a series of curves that form an "S" shape and give the back strength and resilience. To have perfect posture, the curves need to be just right. Some of the main "bad" postural habits you need to look out for are:

- *head pulling back and down*
- *neck pulling too far forward*
- *shoulders hunching up, rounding forward, or pushing too far back*
- *bending forward from the waist*
- *overarching at the lower back*
- *overstiffening the hands and arms*
- *locking at the knees.*

use a deep and powerful form of massage to soften the tissue known as fascia that covers and separates every muscle in the body, and to loosen and stretch muscle and other soft tissues. The aim is to sculpt and realign the body so that it can work with gravity, rather than against it. Rolfing is mainly used to improve posture, treat muscle pain and sports injuries, relieve breathing problems, and improve well-being. Rolfing is inappropriate for people who tend to bruise easily, are very overweight, or have cancer, rheumatoid arthritis, or other inflammatory conditions.

Good posture

Take your shoes off, stand with your feet hip width apart and pointing straight forward, and with your knees soft (slightly bent). Let your shoulders relax down, and allow your arms and hands to hang loosely by your sides. Imagine that you have a wire attached to the top of your head pulling you up.

Keep breathing and imagine your spine lengthening (from your tail bone right up to your neck) as you breathe out, and relaxing as you breathe in. Don't try to flatten the natural curves in your back. Gently tilt your pelvis backward and forward a little until you find the most comfortable position for it.

stress

Stress is a common feature of modern life but means different things to different people. What might be stressful for one person may be experienced as an enjoyable challenge by another. Some stress can be a good thing, giving us extra motivation to carry out an important job well. However, stress isn't always associated with unpleasant situations. Joyful events like a birth, marriage, or start of a new job can be stressful. Stress is only a problem when we have too much of it. For about 1 in 20 people, stress is a severe problem.

What is stress?

The way we respond to acute stress, such as a life-threatening event or danger, is instinctive: We either "fight or flee." This is a throwback to our primitive roots, and our bodies are conditioned to get ready to fight or run away from an enemy.

Several hormones are released from the adrenal glands into the bloodstream in response to acute stress, including adrenaline, norepinephrine, and hydrocortisone. These make the heartbeat stronger and speed up breathing so that more oxygen flows through the body. Blood flow to the brain and muscles increases, so the brain becomes more alert, the muscles contract so they are ready for action, and blood flow is reduced in other parts of the body that aren't needed to survive the emergency, like the digestive tract and skin. The pupils of the eyes dilate to let in more light and become more sensitive, and hearing becomes more keen. The body is on red alert. When we are under chronic stress, our bodies are on constant red alert, and this can lead to physical and emotional symptoms.

Stress refers to the pressures on a person that are in some way felt to be excessive or overwhelming, as well as to the psychological and physical changes that occur in response to those pressures.

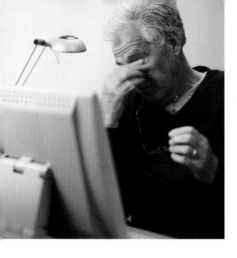

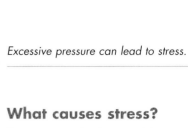

Excessive pressure can lead to stress.

What causes stress?

Stress is not only determined by external events but how we perceive and respond to the events as an individual. Although actors might love performing on stage, a shy person might find it intolerably stressful. Sometimes stress follows on from or is somehow linked to a specific event in a person's life. Death of one's spouse or a close relative, divorce, and imprisonment are considered to be the most stressful events. Injury and illness, job loss or retirement, acute problems with sex, or an illness in a family member come next. Other events that can also cause stress include marriage, a wanted pregnancy, changes in financial status, taking out a mortgage, changing jobs, death of a close friend, or trouble with the in-laws. A person often starts feeling stressed when several potentially stressful events happen close together. If we also have other worries—for example, poor housing, concern about our children's education, or noisy neighbors—a stressful event might be the last straw.

Signs and symptoms of stress

We respond to stress in many ways. Some people experience physical signs and symptoms, such as cold, sweaty palms; a pale face; headaches; back or chest pain; breathlessness or hyperventilation; a lump in the throat; dizziness; palpitations; tiredness; muscle twitching; indigestion; or diarrhea. Alternatively, an existing condition might get worse, such as chronic pain, migraine, asthma, eczema, or irritable bowel syndrome. Some of us might react emotionally in our behavior. We might get more short-tempered, anxious, agitated, depressed, or weepy or we might have difficulty sleeping or poor concentration. Our eating patterns might change, or we might start taking drugs, drinking, or smoking more. Often, someone who is stressed will have several signs and symptoms. Prolonged stress has been implicated in several conditions. Although dermatologists don't believe it can lead to baldness, trichologists (hair specialists) do. As blood flow is reduced to the scalp during the fight-or-flight response, trichologists believe that the hair follicles stop getting the nutrients and oxygen they need, and this can lead to hair loss. Stress hasn't been shown to be an independent cause of cancer, but research has found that women who have experienced a high level of stress and who don't have any intimate emotional social support are more likely to develop breast cancer. Stress has been linked with a depressed immune system, low sperm count and infertility in men, stomach ulcers, high blood pressure, and the initial symptoms of diabetes.

Self-help for stress

One of the most important first steps in managing stress is recognizing it. If two or more of the following apply to you, it is probably time to slow down and learn how to manage stress. Do you:

- regularly sleep for less than 7 hours a night?
- often seem to be in a hurry?
- often have to work under tight deadlines or long hours?
- often feel under pressure at work?
- seem to argue a lot and find relationships difficult?
- rarely have time to relax or sit down to a proper meal?

You can do many things for yourself to help manage stress. The most important one is to lead a healthier life. Try not to smoke, drink alcohol, or take drugs when you are under stress, because addictions such as these can aggravate the symptoms of stress. A good night's sleep (see p.88) and regular exercise (see p.64) can work wonders with helping you have a stress-free day. Eating regularly and healthily (see p.54) is vital to your well-being. Cutting down on drinks like cola, tea, and coffee also helps because caffeine heightens stress.

You can also try changing your daily activities and pastimes. Time management (see p.81) can give you time to unwind. Loneliness and social isolation can make mental stress much harder to deal with. Local support groups can help you feel that you are not alone, and clubs can help meet new friends. Hobbies and pastimes can be an effective way of diverting attention from your worries. Make time every week to do something you enjoy. For some people, spiritual practices and retreats help deal with stress. However, beware of cult groups, based on one charismatic individual, which insist on members isolating themselves from their families and friends.

Coping with stress may involve changing your habits, your relationships, and your attitudes. Try to identify events that are stressful, and rehearse ways to deal with them. Try not to ignore problems hoping they will go away; it is better to confront an issue and make a decision about it. The next section introduces some of the techniques or therapies to help you deal with stress.

Techniques for stress management

Relaxation, mediation, visualization, autogenics, biofeedback, deep breathing (see p.85), tai chi (see p.70), and yoga (see p.114) are all beneficial techniques you can learn. Several complementary therapies have a positive effect on stress and its symptoms, including acupuncture (see p.100), aromatherapy (see p.120), massage (see p.104), and reflexology (see p.112). There are herbal medicines (see p.122) that can help you relax, and doctors may prescribe a drug such as diazepam (Valium) to help with stress. However, these drugs can cause dependence and withdrawal symptoms after a week or two.

Talking to a trained counselor or psychotherapist might help, particularly if you tend to be pessimistic and become stressed by change. Cognitive-behavioral therapy examines your reaction to an event and helps you modify your behavior. A depressed person should always seek medical advice. One of the best ways of avoiding stress is to structure your activities so that you can relax or do something you enjoy. Planning ahead can help to avert panic and give you a sense of control. The following tips should help you manage your time:

• Be realistic about what you can do.
• Learn to be assertive and say "no" so that you don't overcommit yourself.
• Organize your day so that you can avoid rushing.
• Prioritize and make lists, to see what needs to be done today and what can be done the next day or later on.
• Arrive at work early enough to give you time to plan the day's tasks. Delegate jobs if possible.
• Treat each task separately to make the workload seem less overwhelming and help you identify the priorities.
• Make time to relax, have fun, eat well, and exercise.
• Have a good night's sleep (see sleep and insomnia, p.88).

relaxation

techniques

There are many things that you can do to help you relax and unwind at the end of a busy day. You might like to listen to music, read a book, or do some gardening. However, deep relaxation doesn't really happen until the mind is calm and still, the muscles deeply relaxed, and the breathing regular and slow.

Several techniques—such as muscle relaxation, deep abdominal breathing, meditation, and visualization—can help you relax and reduce stress. What's more, they can be performed quite easily with a little practice. Although some techniques can be practiced almost anywhere, complete relaxation is more likely to be achieved in calm surroundings. Pleasant lighting, a minimum of noise (except perhaps some gentle music or a guided-relaxation tape), and no hustle and bustle can really help.

As well as enhancing your feelings of well-being, relaxation has been shown to help treat asthma, irritable bowel syndrome, and chronic pain. Research has also found that it helps to prevent nausea resulting from chemotherapy and helps lower blood pressure. High stress levels do not help recovery from any illness, which is why it is important to achieve a relaxed state when suffering from poor health or recuperating from an illness.

Muscle relaxation

These exercises are designed to allow all the muscles in your body to relax, and to help you clear and focus your mind.

Deep muscle relaxation involves tensing all the muscles in your body at the same time and then letting them go all at once.

• Lie flat on the floor on your back with your legs together and straight, and a blanket under your head and neck for support. Let your body feel heavy, as if it is sinking into the floor and letting go.

• Let your arms fall out, palms upward and about 2 feet (61 centimeters) away from your body. Let your legs fall slightly apart. Close your eyes. Putting a rolled up flannel or something similar over your eyes can help you relax even more.

• Take a deep breath into your lower abdomen (see below for more about deep abdominal breathing), and tense all the muscles in your body as much as you can. As you breathe out, let all the muscles relax.

• Take a few normal breaths, and then repeat the whole process again two or three times.

Progressive muscle relaxation is similar to deep muscle relaxation but involves tensing and relaxing one muscle group at a time. It can be practiced lying down, sitting, or standing up, so it can even be done at work. It also helps you gain more awareness of your body, as it teaches you how the different muscle groups feel when they are contracted.

• With each muscle group, hold the muscles tense or tight for a count of ten, and then slowly relax them. Keep breathing calmly and smoothly the whole time.

• Start with your hands and lower arms by clenching your hands into a fist. Now, move on to your upper arms, again by clenching your hands into fists and then bringing them up to your shoulders by bending at the elbows.

• To work the forehead and face, first frown and relax, then tightly close your eyes and let them go, and finally raise your eyebrows and release them back down again. Next, thrust your jaw forward and relax it. To work the neck, press your chin in, and then release it. With the shoulders, hunch them up, and then let them drop. With the stomach, buttocks, thighs, and legs, tense and relax them each in turn. Finally, flex the feet, and then release them. After you have tensed and relaxed every part of your body, breathe deeply for 5–10 minutes.

Deep abdominal breathing

Also called diaphragmatic breathing, deep abdominal breathing can help you relax and can train you to breathe into your abdomen. Although this is the healthy way to breathe, many of us don't do it. Instead, we breathe into our upper chest and lungs. This can lead to overbreathing (hyperventilation) and many symptoms similar to those of stress (see p.78), such as palpitations, twitchy muscles, and headache. You can tell how you breathe by having someone place their hands lightly on your shoulders. If their hands move up and down when you breathe, you are a chest breather not an abdominal breather. If you are an abdominal breather, when you put your hands on your abdomen, you should feel your abdomen move out as you inhale.

What to do

Lie down on the floor flat on your back, with your legs out straight and your feet in a relaxed position, falling out slightly, and your head and neck supported on a folded blanket. Place one hand on your abdomen, just over your navel, and the other on your chest. Make sure you are comfortable, then close your eyes and concentrate on your breathing without altering it. Breathe in deeply enough to move the hand on your abdomen up, then breathe out so that your hand moves down again. If the hand on your chest moves more than the one on your abdomen, you

At the end of a busy activity, relaxing in a warm bath, scented with a few drops of aromatherapy oil, can be the perfect way to unwind.

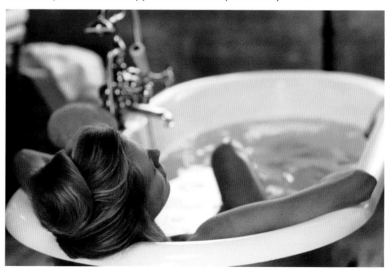

are not breathing deeply enough. Try to practice deep abdominal breathing for about 10 minutes. The more you practice, the sooner your body will learn how to breathe abdominally all the time.

Meditation

Although meditation has been part of many spiritual practices for centuries, it is only recently that researchers have discovered its therapeutic benefits. Meditation aims to clear the mind of all thoughts and induce a relaxed state. To achieve this, focus on one thing, such as a candle flame or some other natural object. Chant a mantra (silently or audibly), or focus on your breathing. If none of these methods work for you, another simple way to meditate is to clear your mind and detach yourself from any thoughts you may have. When a thought appears, imagine that it is drifting by you on a cloud rather than letting yourself get drawn into it.

You can meditate lying down, sitting, or standing up. Sitting is probably best, either on an upright chair or on a cushion on the floor with your back against the wall if necessary. Standing is tiring, and it is easy to fall asleep when lying down. Whatever position you choose, make sure you can be comfortable in it for about 20 minutes. The more still you are, the more effective the meditation will be.

Focusing on the breath

During this type of meditation, you need to breathe in and out normally, without altering your breathing in any way. There are four stages to this meditation, each lasting about 5 minutes, or six rounds of 10 breaths each. You can either use a watch to time yourself or go by instinct. Once you are comfortable, close your eyes.

Stage 1 Breathe in and out and count 1 in your head. Repeat, count 2, and so on up to 10. Then begin at 1 again.

Stage 2 Instead of counting after a breath, count before a breath. For example, count 1 in your head, then breathe in and out, count 2, breathe in, and so on.

Stage 3 Stop counting and focus on the movements and sensations in your chest as you breathe in and out.

Stage 4 Focus your attention on the air moving in and out of your nostrils. It will feel cool as you breathe in and warm as you breathe out.

Visualization

Visualization uses positive thoughts and images to reduce any negative emotions and fears you might have and to enhance your self-image. It can also be used to help you create what you want in life. For example, if you want to be more relaxed, imagining a calm and peaceful environment, such as a beautiful lake, forest glade, or sunny meadow can slow your breathing down and help you feel calmer. It can also enhance your sense of well-being.

Simply lie down and imagine your chosen setting, perhaps with some music in the background to help you with the visualization. There are many guided visualizations now available on tape or CD. Start by creating a clear mental picture of the scene or goal for which you are aiming, then focus on this picture repeatedly. You can do this while lying down quietly, and you can also imagine it for short periods, anytime throughout the day. Remember to repeat affirmations to yourself, such as "I am relaxed and calm."

Autogenics

Autogenic training is a relaxation therapy based on a series of simple mental exercises aimed at increasing passive awareness of your body. It is used to manage stress and relieve its symptoms by switching off the body's fight-or-flight response and switching on its relaxation response. Usually, autogenics is taught as a course, but once you learn it, you can use it anytime.

Autogenic training might not be appropriate for you if you have ever had psychiatric treatment or have a heart or circulatory condition. If this applies to you, consult your doctor first before embarking on a course.

Biofeedback

The aim of biofeedback is to give a person control over his or her body's functions. Biofeedback therapists use machines that allow you to observe how certain bodily functions (such as blood pressure, heart rate, or muscle tension) change in different circumstances. You are then taught how to control or alter these functions using techniques such as relaxation and meditation. Biofeedback can help you control bodily functions in times of stress, which may mean that you can avoid taking drugs for stress-related problems such as high blood pressure or irritable bowel symptoms,

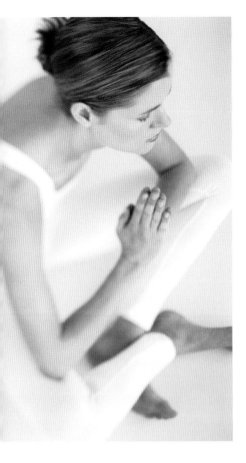

Meditation is a technique that reduces stress and helps you to relax.

or avoid the physical effects of stress or anxiety such as palpitations and breathlessness. You can purchase a biofeedback machine and teach yourself how to use it, but it is probably best to have some sessions with a specialist first.

Hypnotherapy

Hypnotherapy is one of a wide range of techniques that come under the title of mind-body medicine. Hypnosis induces a state of deep relaxation and brings a sense of calm and tranquillity. It is believed to be a useful tool to treat stress-related problems, such as irritable bowel syndrome, insomnia, and anxiety. During hypnotherapy, a person is conscious but accepts suggestions more readily than usual and acts on them more powerfully. Nobody is really sure how hypnotherapy works but one theory is that the left, analytical side of the brain switches off during a hypnotic state, giving the right, creative side a free rein.

A hypnotherapy session usually lasts for between 30 and 90 minutes. While you are under hypnosis, the hypnotherapist may ask you questions to find out the causes of your condition, and then may also take you through procedures and suggestions to relieve your condition.

Different methods are used to induce a hypnotic state, including speaking to you slowly and soothingly and asking you to look at lights or at a pencil held at the limits of your vision. You may also be taught techniques of self-hypnosis to help you manage your condition in your daily life.

sleep and insomnia

We sleep for about a third of our lives. Some people see this as a waste of time, whereas others enjoy the rest it brings. Why we sleep so much is still not completely understood but good sleep is vital for our physical and mental health.

Sleep gives the brain time to organize and store the information it has taken in during the day, and it gives the body a chance to restore and repair itself. Around one in three people living in industrialized societies suffer from severe sleep problems, whereas only about one in five have no sleep disturbances. Everyone else tends to suffer minor but recurring sleep disturbances about one night in seven.

The benefits of sleep

Sleep is essential, and all sorts of problems can arise if we have too little. People who sleep well tend to be healthier and live longer than those who don't. They are also less likely to have accidents—about half of which are due to poor-quality sleep—and they are also more productive. A good night's sleep makes us feel better and happier, whereas a bad one can leave us feeling low and grumpy. Sleep can help us cope with stress and recover from illness.

Researchers have recorded the activity of people's brains while they are sleeping, with some interesting results. Two states of sleep alternate in $1^1/_2$–2 hour cycles: non–rapid eye movement sleep (NREM), or dreamless sleep; and rapid eye movement sleep (REM), or dreaming sleep. Both states are essential to a good night's sleep.

When we first fall asleep, we are in the NREM state, which is a resting phase for the brain. This is when the body repairs and regenerates itself, building bone and muscle and strengthening the immune system. It is this type of sleep that we seem to get less of as we get older. Some researchers believe that we might delay the aging process if we could find ways of maintaining this state of sleep.

When we go into the REM state of sleep, the activity of the brain increases and we dream. The body rests during this cycle and muscles are relaxed. Only the eyes under the eyelids move from side to side, hence the name "rapid eye movement" sleep. The importance of REM sleep is not fully understood. Some experts think it acts as a sort of safety valve, giving our brains time to work through emotional issues. Others think it is important in terms of memory and learning.

Sleep and traditional Chinese medicine

Chinese medicine asserts that if we wake up at the same hour every night for any length of time, it could indicate a physical problem or imbalance. For example, they believe that waking at about 4 o'clock in the morning is associated with lung conditions such as asthma.

The optimal amount of sleep

Some adults seem to manage on 4 to 5 hours of sleep, although research suggests this is rare. Researchers have conflicting opinions on what is the ideal amount of sleep for an adult; some think we need as much as 9 to 10 hours a night, others claim that 6 hours is the minimum and 7 to 8 hours is plenty. Generally, we need more sleep the younger we are: Babies need about 15 hours every day, children between ages 5 and 15 need about 9 hours, adolescents require about 11 hours, and the elderly need about 6 hours. Whenever we are ill, we tend to need more sleep than usual.

Insomnia

It is perfectly normal to wake up in the night and the older we get, the longer we may wake up for. A problem occurs when we are unable to fall back to sleep again quickly. However, research into sleeping patterns suggests that even people with insomnia or those who sleep lightly or irregularly get more sleep than they think they do.Nonetheless, sleep deprivation is a a serious matter. It is an important risk factor predicting death, and two thirds of us do not get adequate sleep. Sleep loss is cumulative and results in decreased cognitive functions, increased susceptibility to illness, behavioral abnormalities, and accidents.

Understanding the cause

Anxiety, stress, and overwork can make relaxing difficult and so lead to insomnia. An emotional crisis such as divorce or bereavement can also make sleeping difficult. Insomnia can also be a sign of emotional illness like depression, or it can be caused by pain from a physical condition such as arthritis.

Treating the problem

The most important first step to treating insomnia is to find the cause of it. Relaxation, meditation, and deep-breathing techniques (see p.83) can help you unwind if the problem is due to stress. Prescribed drugs are sometimes given for a few days to help someone through a crisis or a time of great emotional stress. However, they can lead to dependence if taken for more than a few weeks. Little specific research has been done to measure the effectiveness of complementary therapies, although acupuncture, aromatherapy, massage, and yoga are all known to help people relax. Herbal medicine (see p.122) can also be useful, and several herbs are available to help you sleep, including hops, lemon balm, orange blossom, passion flower, peppermint, and valerian.

Snoring and sleep apnea

Snoring can be more of a problem for partners than the snorers themselves. However, it can also be associated with a more serious condition known as sleep apnea, where the affected person stops breathing for short periods many times during the night. This leads to repeated waking, which can disturb sleep, and also depletes the body of oxygen. During the day, a person with sleep apnea may feel exhausted and irritable. Sleep apnea can be caused by a blocked airway or because the nerves that stimulate breathing are faulty. It is most common in overweight men ages 30 to 50.

Jet lag, night shifts, and melatonin

If we disturb our regular sleep patterns by taking long-distance flights or working irregular shifts, we can experience symptoms such as tiredness, hunger or loss of appetite, headache, irritability, and lack of concentration. These symptoms result from your body and brain telling you it is time to sleep. Supplements of melatonin, a substance produced in the brain in response to light, have been shown to be an effective treatment for jet lag or sleep disturbance from shift work. Research shows that it may help to shorten the time it takes us to adapt to a new pattern of sleep and wakefulness, but long-term trials on melatonin's safety and effectiveness have not been completed. Low levels of light causes decreased melatonin production, which in turn can create depression, but full spectrum light therapy can produce an improvement after a few hours.

TIPS FOR A GOOD NIGHT'S SLEEP

Try to ensure your bedroom is quiet (or wear ear plugs), well ventilated, and not too hot or cold. Have a regular bedtime, and get up at the same time each morning. Also, keep the following points in mind.

- *Try not to nap in the daytime.*
- *Avoid caffeinated stimulants (like tea, coffee, hot chocolate, or cola) during the evening.*
- *Avoid drinking too much alcohol. While alcohol may help you get to sleep, it can also cause you to wake very early.*
- *Avoid large meals late in the evening, but don't go to bed hungry.*
- *Try having warm milk or a whole-grain biscuit just before going to sleep.*
- *Avoid working, watching television, or having intense or difficult conversations late into the evening.*
- *Exercise regularly.*
- *Have a warm bath just before you go to bed.*
- *Use aromatherapy oils such as lavender in an oil burner.*
- *Save the bedroom for sleep (and sex).*

skin care

How we feel about our skin has a huge psychological impact on us, because it is what other people see. The skin is not just an outer covering for the body, it is a living organ, the largest organ in the body, and it plays a major part in helping the body to rid itself of waste products. It also helps keep us cool, is waterproof, stretches, and is highly sensitive to touch.

The outer layers of the skin are constantly falling off and being replaced: About 10 billion dead skin cells fall off our bodies every 24 hours. The skin contains sweat glands, oil glands, hair follicles, collagen (support tissue) and elastic fibers, nerves, and blood vessels. Healthy skin relies on a good blood flow to bring it nutrients and oxygen. Our skin is the first organ to show signs of aging. As we age, the skin loses its elasticity and begins to thin, as collagen and elastic fibers are lost. It tends to dry out, especially in women around the time of menopause (see p.38).

Dealing with wrinkles

You cannot stop wrinkles from developing, because they are part of the normal aging process. Creams, ointments, and lotions can all help keep your skin looking healthy, mainly by keeping it moist. However, spending vast amounts of money on expensive beauty products is not the answer to beautiful, wrinkle-free skin. Rose water and glycerin from your local pharmacist are just as good as expensive products but a lot cheaper, and they can be used to cleanse and moisturize your skin. It is the way you treat your skin every day, plus careful attention to your diet, general health, and well-being that is more important. The skin is a mirror of your general health and reflects what is going on in your mind and body. Some factors can increase the amount of wrinkles you get and speed up the skin-aging process. These include exposure to the sun, smoking, excess alcohol, prolonged stress, lack of sleep, illness, and internal

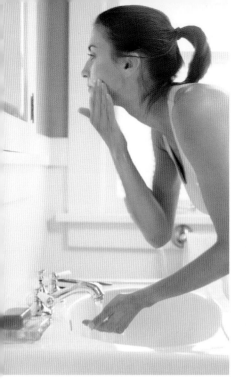

Regular skin cleansing is essential to keep it looking healthy.

pollution from too many chemicals in your diet. To help keep your skin looking young and healthy for as long as possible, don't smoke, cut down on alcohol, drink lots of water, wear a high-SPF sunscreen and a hat when you are out in the sun, try to avoid too much stress, get enough sleep (see p.88), and eat well.

Other things you can do to help prevent wrinkles are general exercise (see p.64), facial exercises (see p.94), yoga (see p.114), relaxation (see p.82), and diet (see p.54). Many dermatologists believe that sloughing off dead skin cells (exfoliation) can stimulate cell reproduction. When men shave, they remove dead cells from their face with hair, which may be why men's skin ages less quickly than women's. The female hormone, estrogen (see p.38), taken as hormone replacement therapy after menopause, may help reduce wrinkles by improving the amount of collagen in the skin, increasing its water content, and stimulating blood flow. Certain essential oils (see p.120) are reputed to be good for aging skin, such as sandalwood, rose, myrrh, frankincense, lavender, and clary sage. Facial massage (see p.107), acupressure, and acupuncture (see p.100) are thought to help prevent wrinkles by improving blood flow to the skin and increasing facial muscle tone, though this is not confirmed. Another option is surgery (see p.138), including facelifts and chemosurgery.

Eating for better skin

A balanced diet is vital. Deficiency in any nutrient will show up on your skin. Certain vitamins and minerals (see p.58) are especially important. The three most important nutrients are vitamin A, which is vital to the general health of our skin; vitamin C, without which the body cannot carry out self-renewal; and zinc, which promotes repair and healing. The following vitamins and minerals may be benefit the skin:

- The antioxidants—vitamins A, C, and E, as well as copper, manganese, selenium, and zinc—can all help keep you looking younger.
- Vitamin A and B-complex vitamins may help to remove age spots.
- Thiamine, riboflavin, and pyridoxine may help to prevent premature aging.
- Vitamin C may help prevent stretch marks, easy bruising, and broken veins.
- Zinc may be good for stretch marks and sagging skin.

Some "super foods" are reputed to be good for the skin: carrots, watercress, avocado, melon, strawberries, pumpkin seeds, sprouted seeds, millet, and oats.

Doing facial exercises

One of the best ways to help stop your face from aging is to do facial exercises every day. They can tone facial muscles, improve blood flow to your skin, and help to reduce sagging and wrinkling. They are best done slowly and steadily. You can also use machines that passively exercise your face. Do the forehead exercise without any face cream but make sure you put moisturizer on for the eye and chin exercises; otherwise you may increase the depth of lines you already have.

Forehead Slowly lift your forehead up and open your eyes wider and wider, in controlled steps, for a count of 5–10. Hold for a count of 5 and then slowly release in 5–10 steps. Repeat five times.

Eyes Place your elbows on a table. With your index fingers, press two pieces of folded tissue over the "crows feet" areas next to your eyes. Lower your chin to your chest and, keeping it there, look straight ahead. Then, in 5–10 definite steps, bring your bottom eyelids up to your upper ones, and hold them closed for a count of 5. All the time, work against the pressure of your fingers. Lower the lids, again in 5–10 definite steps, and rest for a count of 4. Do this three times, then repeat without any pressure.

Chin and cheeks Smile with your mouth closed, then push your lower jaw forward as far as possible. Hold it there, then move your jaw from side to side five times. Repeat this 10 times. Next, smile as hard as you can with your mouth closed and the corners of your mouth turned up. At the same time, try to pull your lips into an **O** shape. Hold this for 5 seconds, and repeat five times. Finally, tilt your head backward slightly. Draw your mouth into a tight **O** shape, turn your mouth into a downward smile, back to the **O** shape, and so on. Repeat this movement ten times.

Skin cancer

Skin cancer is one of the most common cancers in the world. Exposure to the sun is the biggest risk factor. Getting sunburned on a short vacation is more dangerous than regular, moderate exposure to the sun. The fairer your skin, the bigger your risk. To prevent skin cancer, avoid excessive exposure to the sun. If you have to be out in the sun for exercise, wear high-SPF sunscreens, and cover up your body. If you have a lump, ulcer, or mole that worries you, see your doctor. Taking extra doses of vitamins C, E and beta carotene before sun exposure may protect against sun damage.

Caring for nails

Nail splitting, weakness, and breakage are all caused by wear and tear, prolonged contact with water, or a diet lacking vitamins or minerals. Biting your nails can also weaken them. If you have split or broken nails, it is unlikely you need medical attention unless you feel unwell. However, nail problems can be a symptom of fungal infection, psoriasis, eczema, or a more serious condition such as heart disease. Consult your doctor if you are concerned that you might have one of these conditions. White spots on the nails suggest a zinc or vitamin B_6 deficiency, whereas pale, flat, thin, and dry nails can suggest iron deficiency. Low stomach acid has been associated with brittle nails. For healthy strong nails, eat a balanced diet of foods high in sulfur, iron, zinc, calcium, and vitamins A, B, and C. If your nails are very weak, try a vitamin and mineral supplement for a few months. Wear rubber gloves when you wash dishes. The tissue salt silicea (see p.129) may strengthen split or broken nails.

Doing daily exercises for hands and nails

1. Stretch your fingers out fully, then clench them into a tight fist. Open and close your hands quickly like this at least ten times.

2. Close one of your hands into a fist, then wrap the other hand around it and squeeze tightly. Do this five times, then repeat on the other hand.

3. Relax the fingers on one hand. With the other hand, hold the end of each finger in turn and gently pull it. Repeat on the other hand.

4. With the fleshy pad of the thumb of one hand, massage the palm of the other, using small circular movements. Repeat on the other hand.

5. End by gently shaking out your hands.

healthy
hair

Healthy hair depends not only on what is put on it but also on our mental and physical state. If we have a well-balanced diet, are unstressed and keep fit, we are more likely to have beautiful hair. Other factors such as hormones, medications and surgeries may also play important roles in maintaining healthy hair.

Hair loss

The most common type of hair loss is known as male pattern baldness (androgenous alopecia), which is the baldness that many men, and some women, typically get as they grow older. It starts with a receding hairline, then thinning on top of the head until most of the head is bald. About one in 20 men have started balding by the age 20. This type of balding is not caused by hair loss but by a change in the type of hair that grows on the head. Instead of the coarse, thick "terminal hairs" that usually grow during the adult years, small, colorless, soft "vellus hairs" start growing. This type of hair also grows on the insides of the arms and is virtually invisible to the naked eye. Half of all men with this type of baldness have inherited it. Other risk factors include age and excess testosterone. This male hormone stops hair follicles from producing terminal hairs. Some experts believe that eating foods containing high levels of male hormones (such as brewer's yeast, wheat germ, and peanut oil) can increase the risk of male pattern baldness, but this is a controversial issue.

Another type of hair loss, known as general baldness (or alopecia), can affect men and women equally. Various dietary factors are thought to contribute to this type of hair loss, such as too much or too little vitamin A, a shortage of vitamin B_{12} and iron, and intake of oral contraceptives. It can also be caused by a shock or stress on the body, such as a high prolonged fever, a crash diet, pregnancy and childbirth, certain drugs like anticancer drugs, prolonged periods of mental stress, or thyroid deficiency. With male baldness, little can be done to restore terminal hair once it has stopped growing. However, treating the scalp to improve the health of the hair follicles might help if done at the first signs of hair loss. Taking supplements of biotin and inositol may help prevent male baldness, but good evidence is lacking. Some prescription drugs can stimulate hair growth, such as inhibitors that block testosterone action; minoxidil (Rogaine); and retinoic acid (a derivative of vitamin A). These treatments must be taken continuously. Once the drug is stopped, the hair is lost again; within 3 months it will be as it was before treatment. Hair transplants are also an option. For general hair loss, eating a healthy and balanced diet, possibly taking a multivitamin and mineral supplement, and reducing your stress levels (see p.78) are all important. The healthier you are, the healthier your hair will be. Eating oily fish and regularly taking supplements of fish oils or flax seed oil may be beneficial. Arnica cream, a homeopathic remedy (see p.126) may help, but this has not been thoroughly researched. A regular, vigorous scalp massage with rosemary oil in a base of almond, olive, or jojoba oil is reported to increase blood circulation and bring nutrients and oxygen to the hair follicles. Rubbing in lavender or thyme oil in a base may stimulate hair growth. Rub into the scalp once or twice a week, and leave on for a few hours before washing.

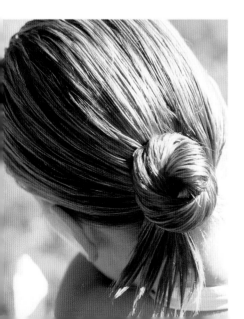

Herbal infusion for hair loss

1. Place $3/4$ oz (25 g) of dried rosemary, sage, or stinging nettle or $2 1/2$ oz (75 g) of fresh herbs in a teapot.
2. Add 17 oz (500 ml) of boiling hot water.
3. Put the lid on, and leave for 10 minutes.
4. Strain and store in a cool place.
This should produce enough for 3–4 rinses.

Shining, healthy hair depends on our physical and mental state.

therapies

So far, we've looked at the different dietary and lifestyle measures that can help you "beat the years" and improve your health and general well-being. Complementary and conventional medical approaches have previously been mentioned—and here we look more closely at these different approaches.

More and more people are using complementary therapies along with conventional medicine to treat illnesses, to stay well, and to replace conventional treatment when it has failed to help or has caused unpleasant side effects. As with conventional medicine, you can use elements of many complementary therapies to help yourself, in addition to consulting a qualified practitioner of a particular therapy. The next few pages explore the main therapies available, the conditions that they might be helpful for, and the elements of the therapies you can self-administer to help stay youthful.

Treating the whole person

Historically, the approaches of conventional and complementary medicine have always been different. Conventional medicine was developed on the basis that every sign and symptom has a specific cause that can be treated. It typically uses drugs and/or surgery to treat the parts of the body affected by a disease.

The difference with complementary therapies is that they tend to be holistic and based on the belief that the mind, body, and spirit are inseparable. Practitioners attempt to treat the whole person and to tailor treatments to the individual, not simply hand out formulas for specific symptoms. Over time, the ideas of the holistic approach have made their way into conventional medicine.

There are other overlaps between complementary and conventional medicine and some techniques that complementary medical practitioners use, conventional medical practitioners also use. Many physiotherapists use acupuncture techniques to relieve pain, or manipulation techniques to relieve back problems similar to those used by osteopaths and chiropractors. Many general practitioners use homeopathic remedies and herbal medicines. Massage and aromatherapy are widely practiced by nurses.

A discipline called mind-body medicine is now beginning to flourish in conventional circles. There is also a move to put conventional and complementary medicine under the umbrella term *integrative medicine*.

Using the body's energy

As well as treating disease once it is already present in an individual, conventional medicine also aims to prevent disease, and concentrates on lifestyle and dietary measures. For example, there is an ongoing search for a treatment that can prevent the onset of the symptoms of aging.

Complementary and alternative medicine goes beyond preventing disease because it focuses on stimulating the body's innate self-healing properties. Many complementary and alternative therapies are based on the idea that a life force or vital energy exists in all of us. In various ways, these therapies purport to tap into this energy and help the body to use it in a more productive way.

The most well-established complementary therapies in the Western world are acupuncture, herbal medicine, homeopathy, osteopathy, and chiropractic. Aromatherapy, massage, naturopathy, reflexology, yoga, Ayurveda, and traditional Chinese medicine are also popular. Surveys suggest that the most common conditions for which people seek complementary therapies are arthritis, back pain, headaches and other types of pain, allergic conditions (such as eczema, asthma, and hay fever), feelings of poor health, anxiety and smoking, menstrual and menopausal problems, digestive disorders, and high blood pressure. Most people who seek help are between ages 40 and 60 and have had their problem for more than a year.

As complementary therapies are widely gaining acceptance, it is important to gain answers to questions such as "What sort of evidence is there to show that they work?" and "How safe are they?" These standard questions must be answered before they are given a license for use.

acupuncture

Acupuncture is a part of traditional Chinese medicine (TCM) that has been practiced for thousands of years. It involves the insertion of fine needles into specific points on the body. TCM is comprised of acupuncture, chinese herbal medicine, and qigong, and is used to treat a wide range of illnesses. TCM is a holistic approach to building health and treating illness, by improving physical, emotional, and spiritual well-being.

What is acupuncture?

TCM acupuncture embraces a philosophy that is different from that of conventional medicine. According to TCM theory, we all have qi, which means energy or "life force," flowing through our bodies. Our health and well-being is said to rely on the smooth and balanced flow of qi through a series of channels (meridians) that lie beneath the skin. Illness, on the other hand, is thought to occur because of too much, too little, or blocked qi. Inserting fine needles into specific points, known as acupuncture points, on the meridians is believed to stimulate the body's own healing responses and help restore its natural balance. Sometimes pressure, sound, electricity or lasers, rather than needles, are used on the points. In some conditions the acupuncture points may be warmed using a technique called moxibustion. TCM treatment aims to improve your overall well-being as well as the symptoms of your condition. People often find that acupuncture can lead to increased energy levels, better sleep, and a sense of good health, as well as helping with their specific problem.

Conventional health professionals are also using acupuncture techniques. However, many physicians tend to apply the techniques on the basis of a conventional medical diagnosis, believing that acupuncture may work by stimulating the nerves in skin and muscle to produce various effects on the body's hormones, nervous system, muscle tone, circulation, and immune system. These treatments tend to focus on relieving specific symptoms.

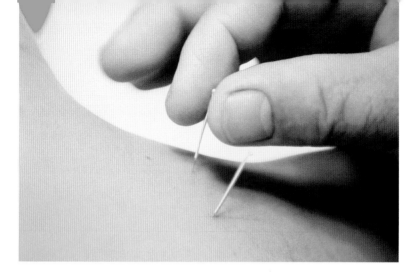

TCM practitioners believe that yin and yang are opposite but complementary forces. Their perfect balance in the body is essential for good health.

Who is acupuncture for?

Acupuncture can be safely given to anyone, young or old, although acupressure rather than needles may be preferred for babies and young children. Some people have acupuncture for specific symptoms or conditions (such as anxiety, arthritis, asthma, or back pain), whereas others have acupuncture to prevent general ill health, to strengthen their constitution, or to help them feel well, even though they are not ill in the conventional medical sense. Acupuncture can even be used during pregnancy, but some of the points must be avoided.

Some evidence now shows that acupuncture works for chronic lower back pain, migraine, dental pain, and nausea and vomiting during pregnancy or after surgery or chemotherapy. Evidence also indicates that it helps conditions such as arthritis, neck pain, menstrual pain, premenstrual tension, and menopausal symptoms, anxiety, allergies such as asthma and hay fever, irritable bowel syndrome, and some drug problems. Acupuncture may also work for other conditions, but further evidence is needed. Some TCM practitioners claim acupuncture works for wrinkles, hair loss, and obesity, but little evidence supports its efficacy in these areas.

Acupuncture needles are very fine, so people usually just feel a slight prick; they do not hurt like needles used to give injections or draw blood. Once a needle has been inserted, it is usually left in place for about 15–20 minutes. While the needle is in place, you may not feel anything or you may feel a tingling or dull ache around the needle. Some TCM acupuncturists try to bring on a sensation called "de qi" at the point of the needle by moving (manipulating) the needle after it has been inserted. This may cause an unpleasant feeling, but most people feel relaxed and often sleep during a treatment.

What happens at an acupuncture session?

At your first acupuncture session, the practitioner will probably spend up to an hour talking to you about your symptoms, possible treatments, medical history, family history, current living and working conditions, diet and digestive system, emotions, and sleeping patterns. A TCM acupuncturist will also feel your pulse and look at your tongue to assess your qi and your yin and yang. A fast pulse is said to result from too much heat in the body, whereas a red tongue with no coating is caused by a yin deficiency.

The acupuncturist uses all this information to work out the best treatment, often choosing 5–10 body points to needle, out of the 500 or so that are known. Sometimes ear acupuncture is used, especially to treat drug addictions or to relieve stress or insomnia. Your acupuncturist might also give you dietary advice, exercise suggestions, or Chinese herbs to supplement your treatment.

At subsequent sessions, the acupuncturist will probably spend 10–15 minutes talking to you before deciding which acupuncture points to use. Most people with an acute problem require at least three treatments at weekly intervals, although how many acupuncture treatments an individual will need can vary. Those with a chronic condition might need to go weekly for about five sessions, then twice weekly for a few sessions, then monthly. Most people should notice some change after five acupuncture treatments.

Is acupuncture safe?

Minor effects of acupuncture include local superficial bruising, fainting, feeling sick, a local reaction where the needle has been, or pain. Rare but serious adverse effects include infection, a punctured lung, and spinal cord injury. Such effects usually result from a poorly trained practitioner, so it is important to go to a properly trained and registered acupuncturist (see organizations on p.140).

Acupressure to boost your energy

If you feel tired and sluggish a lot of the time, it could be that your qi is depleted or blocked. Try giving yourself acupressure everyday on the following three points. Simply apply pressure with your thumb or fingertip to these points and hold for about 2 minutes. As you do this, imagine the depression you are making is filling up with qi. Work on each point on both sides of the body.

St36 This point is on the outside of the shin, 4 fingerwidths below the knee. To find it, keep your leg straight, then lay the index finger of the opposite hand along the lower edge of your kneecap. Next, lay the rest of your fingers down side by side. The point is located where the little fingertip falls, just on the outside of the shinbone. If you run your index finger gently over this area, you should also be able to feel a slight dip where the point is.

Sp6 This point is on the inside of the shin, 4 fingerwidths above the ankle. To find this point, bend your leg slightly, and lay the little finger of the same hand next to your inner anklebone. Next, lay the rest of your fingers down side by side. The point is located where the index fingertip falls, just behind your shinbone. This point is often quite painful to pressure. **Warning:** Do not use this point if you are pregnant because it can induce labor.

Liv4 This point is found on the back of the hand, at the end of the crease made between your thumb and index finger when you bring them together. **Warning:** Do not use this point if you are pregnant because it can induce labor.

Qigong

Qigong, or "energy work," is an ancient Chinese system of movement, meditation, and breathing techniques. Its aim is to improve the circulation of qi and so promote health and well-being. It can be practiced by anyone and is used in China for diseases of old age, tiredness, stress, muscle and joint problems, heart disease, high blood pressure, and much more. Research has shown that qigong can have beneficial effects on strength, health, and longevity. One study found that qigong—combining relaxation, breathing exercises, massage, and a walking exercise—increases the blood levels of superoxide dismutase, which is a natural body chemical that attacks harmful free radicals and promotes a healthy immune system. It may work in this way to promote good health and energy levels in older people.

massage

Massage is the application of pressure to the soft tissues
of the body: the skin, muscles, tendons, and ligaments.
Therapeutic massage has probably been around for as long
as humans. Paintings in Egyptian tombs show people being
massaged, and ancient Chinese and Indian manuscripts
refer to massage techniques to treat diseases. What's more,
we all instinctively massage ourselves when we hurt
something or have a pain.

What types of massage are available?

The main types of massage include Swedish massage (also known as classical or
European massage); Oriental types of massage such as Thai, marma (Indian), tuina
(Chinese), and shiatsu (Japanese) massage; Rosen Method Bodywork (mind/body),
and sports massage. Different massage techniques have also been incorporated
into other therapies, such as physiotherapy and osteopathy (see p.108) and in other
types of bodywork, such as rolfing (see p.76). Depending on the techniques used,
massage can relax, strengthen, and stimulate the body.

How do massage techniques differ?

Swedish massage forms the basis of massage techniques used in the West today. This
type of massage was developed by studying the anatomy of the body, and it involves
four main techniques. Effleurage, or stroking, is a smooth, gentle action where the
hands glide rhythmically over the skin, following the direction of the muscle fibers. It is
used all over the body to relax tense muscles and improve circulation. Pétrissage, or
kneading of the skin and soft tissue by squeezing and releasing it, stretches and relaxes
the muscles and is particularly used on fleshy areas. It helps to break up knots in the
muscles and tense spots. Frottage, or friction, involves applying deep pressure with the
thumbs to a specific spot to release tension in the muscles around the spine and

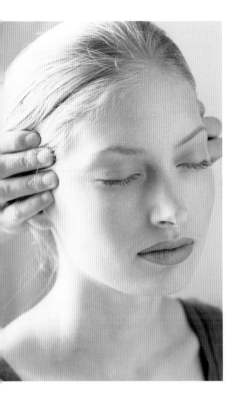

A head massage can help relieve stress and tension headaches.

shoulders. Tapotement, percussion or chopping, with the sides of the hands, is used to stimulate the body, and tone and strengthen the muscles.

Oriental types of massage tend to work on specific body points such as acupuncture points and aim to move energy in the body. Some massage therapists use aromatic oils during their treatments (see aromatherapy on p.120).

What happens during a massage?

A Swedish massage may include a full-body massage, with or without a facial massage, or just a neck and shoulder massage. For a full-body massage, you usually undress down to your underwear, although this isn't compulsory. The therapist usually uses towels to cover the parts of your body not being worked on. Massage therapists use an oil, or sometimes body lotion or talcum powder, to help their hands glide more easily over your skin. The length of a massage session varies, but a full-body massage takes about an hour, $1^1/_2$ hours if the face is included. Other types of massage also take about an hour. The pressure from some massage techniques can be temporarily uncomfortable, but if it is unpleasant, simply ask the massage therapist to ease the pressure. You shouldn't feel persistent pain during a massage and, if you do, stop the treatment immediately.

Does it work?

Scientific trials investigating how massage might work have shown that it generally helps with relaxation, can increase your sense of well-being, helps muscles relax, increases blood flow locally, and increases your pain threshold. However, do any of these effects help people with health problems? Encouraging evidence shows that massage helps to relieve back pain, chronic constipation, and pressure sores, but more studies are needed to confirm this. Evidence that sports massage can prevent muscle injury during vigorous exercise is lacking, and little scientific evidence shows that massage helps to relieve musculoskeletal pain, although there is plenty of anecdotal evidence.

Several clinical trials have found that massage can help relieve anxiety and depression in people who are ill, such as young people with rheumatoid arthritis, children with cystic fibrosis, and patients being treated for cancer. Clinical trials have also found that massage can reduce labor pain, help children with asthma breathe more easily, and help premature babies, heart and stroke patients, and people suffering from AIDS.

Is it safe?

Although massage is safe when carried out by a well-qualified therapist, it should not be used in certain situations. You should not have a massage if you have a serious heart condition, and you should seek medical advice before having a massage if you have a blood clot (thrombosis), varicose veins or inflammation of the veins (phlebitis), a fever, acute arthritis, a severe back problem, an infected skin condition, cancer, HIV or AIDS, epilepsy, or a serious psychiatric illness.

You should also not be massaged on the abdomen, legs, or feet during the first 3 months of pregnancy, and it is best to ask your doctor's advice about massage at other times during pregnancy. You should generally not massage directly over bruises, swellings, or inflamed, infected, or injured parts of the body.

Shiatsu massage and do-in

Shiatsu is based on traditional Chinese medicine principles and uses the same theories of energy and meridians as acupressure (see p.103). Shiatsu was developed in Japan early in the twentieth century. The aims of shiatsu are to diagnose and treat diseases by using pressure applied with the elbows, hands, and fingers. This technique is believed to stimulate the body's own healing powers, remove toxins, and promote general good health.

Although little scientific research has been carried out on shiatsu, it is used to treat various conditions from arthritis and migraines to digestive problems and asthma. Practitioners often teach their patients self-help exercises to maintain good health, which are known as do-in. These exercises have elements of shiatsu and acupressure, and involve stretching exercises, tapping and pressure on acupressure points, breathing techniques, and meditation. Carrying out do-in daily is thought to promote relaxation, tone skin and muscles, improve circulation and flexibility, and improve clarity of thinking.

Indian head massage

Used in Ayurvedic medicine, Indian head massage was thought to keep hair healthy, shiny, and thick by improving blood flow to the scalp and relaxing the muscles of the scalp. Although the effectiveness of this technique has not been scientifically studied, it is certainly relaxing and can help to relieve anxiety and stress.

Face and head massage

If you are feeling stressed or have a tension headache, a head and face massage can really help you unwind. You can either do it yourself or get a willing friend or partner to do it for you. Simply follow the steps below.

• Always have clean hands when massaging.
• Warm your hands by rubbing them together or by soaking them in warm water.
• Lie down and close your eyes.
• Using the flats of your fingers, massage your forehead, starting in the center and moving outward in long, firm strokes.
• End at your temples, massaging them in small circular movements with your fingertips. Repeat these movements several times.
• Next, using similar strokes, massage along your cheekbones, cheeks, and jaw.
• Using your fingertips, massage in small circles just below the ear end of your cheekbones and a couple of inches below this, at your jaw joints.
• Finally, starting at the crown of your head, massage your scalp with your fingertips, using ever-larger circles until you reach your hairline

This massage should take about 15 minutes. Rest for a couple of minutes afterward before getting up slowly.

osteopathy and chiropractic

Osteopathy and chiropractic are both manipulation-based therapies that have their roots as far back as 400 B.C. The therapies have much in common, but they also have many differences. Osteopaths lay equal emphasis on the joints and surrounding soft tissue such as the muscles, tendons, and ligaments, whereas chiropractors focus more on the joints of the spine and the nervous system.

Osteopathy and chiropractic look at the whole body system, which they believe can heal itself if allowed to. They believe that many health problems can be traced to poor posture and to misalignment of muscles and joints, particularly the spine, and that improving body structure and correcting misalignment restores health. The cause of misalignment is usually considered to be external, such as a fall, twist, or jolt, which may have happened years before or may result from long-term poor posture. Manipulation is used not only to correct joint spinal dysfunction but also to augment general body function, which is mediated through the nervous system, circulation, and lymphatics.

What happens during osteopathy and chiropractic?

The first session with an osteopath or chiropractor usually lasts about an hour with subsequent sessions lasting about 30 minutes. At the first session, you will be asked for your medical history, and then you will undergo a thorough physical examination with you sitting, standing, walking, and perhaps carrying out other movements. Your reflexes will be tested and your blood pressure measured. Some chiropractors also use X rays and other standard medical tests to help them make a diagnosis.

Treatment takes place with you lying down in various positions, usually with your outer clothes removed. Sometimes a chiropractor will wait until the second session before starting treatment so that the X-ray results are available. Chiropractors mainly use manipulation on the spinal column and pelvic area, and this tends to consist of short, rapid, forceful movements called high-velocity thrusts, which are designed to realign the spine. When a manipulation is performed, you may hear a click. However, there is a wide variety of non-forceful techniques that are now commonly used.

Osteopaths use various techniques, from massage and stretching of soft tissues to rhythmic joint movements, manipulation, and other techniques on the back and various parts of the body. Although they also carry out high-velocity thrusts on the spine, these form a much smaller part of treatment than in chiropractic. Osteopaths may use only gentle release techniques with some patients, particularly children and older people. These are called "muscle energy techniques," during which you work against resistance provided by the osteopath to release tension in specific muscles. Osteopaths may also carry out cranial manipulation (see p. 111). Your osteopath or chiropractor may show you exercises to do at home and suggest ways you can improve your posture. Many practitioners also give nutritional advice, and some osteopaths are trained in naturopathy (see p. 130).

What are they used for?

Both osteopathy and chiropractic are mainly used to treat back and neck problems. In addition, they are often used to treat other problems that may stem from misalignment of the spine, such as headaches, migraines, vertigo, and tinnitus. Some practitioners also treat arthritic conditions, sports injuries, digestive problems, breathing disorders, and menstrual problems. The main aims of osteopathy and chiropractic are to reduce pain and inflammation, improve movement, and improve general health.

Do they work?

Osteopathy and chiropractic are two complementary therapies most accepted by conventional medical practitioners. Osteopaths are fully licensed and function as conventional doctors in the United States, whereas chiropractors have a more limited role. Many studies have shown that chiropractic is effective in treating lower back pain. Several reviews of trials have looked at spinal manipulation and mobilization for lower back pain in general and one review specifically looked at osteopathy. These reviews suggest that manipulation and mobilization techniques—whether done by an osteopath, chiropractor, physiotherapist, or a doctor—provide short-term relief of pain and improvement in mobility. Although fewer trials of manipulation and mobilization techniques for neck pain exist, clinical experience clearly demonstrates the effectiveness of manipulation in the thoracic and cervical areas in order to relieve neck pain.

Are they safe?

The most serious potential risks with osteopathy and chiropractic are stroke and spinal cord injury after neck manipulation. It has been shown that these injuries occur in approximately one in a million adjustments. More common but less serious adverse effects include mild pain or discomfort at the site of manipulation, mild headaches, and tiredness. These usually disappear within 24 hours of the treatment.

There are some conditions where forceful manipulation carries increased risk, such as with severe osteoporosis of the spine, osteoarthritis of the neck, and pregnancy. Both osteopaths and chiropractors are trained to check patients for these

Osteopathy and chiropractic are both used to treat back and neck problems, with the aim of reducing pain and improving movement in the area.

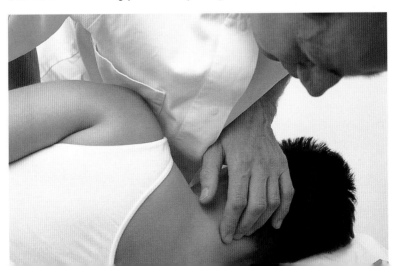

and other risk factors. Even if you have one of these conditions, other more gentle manipulative techniques may be suitable.

Cranial osteopathy

Also called cranial manipulation, carnial osteopathy involves gentle and subtle techniques of manipulation on the skull. Cranial osteopaths believe that childbirth, an accident, or long-term muscle tension can cause compression of the skull, which can affect the way cerebrospinal fluid flows in the spine and around the brain, causing illness. They claim that gently manipulating the bones of the skull can restore it to its natural shape and correct the flow of cerebrospinal fluid. Little clinical research has been done on cranial osteopathy, although it is widely used on babies, young children, and older people.

Craniosacral therapy developed from cranial osteopathy and is similar to it, but it differs in that it believes the rhythmic flow of cerebrospinal fluid affects every cell in the body.

McTimoney and McTimoney-Corley chiropractic

Two variations of chiropractic that use more gentle manipulation techniques than conventional chiropractic are McTimoney and McTimoney-Corley chiropratic. The practitioners of these types of chiropractic also put more emphasis on a holistic approach to ill health and on self-help. Like cranial osteopathy, these techniques tend to be more suitable for babies, young children, and older people.

Correct posture

Squat down with a straight back when lifting an object from the floor or when you are gardening. As you lift the object, hold it close to your body and let your legs take the weight. Never bend at the waist or twist to lift something.

When pushing a heavy object, do so by leaning your back against it and using your legs to do the pushing. Never push it in front of you with your arms.

When carrying heavy loads, use two bags of equal weight, one in each hand, to balance the load.

When driving or sitting, always sit up straight and make sure your lower back is supported by the chair's back. Avoid crossing your legs when sitting.

reflexology

Reflexology, sometimes called reflex zone therapy, involves the massage of certain points on the feet and, less often, the hands. Reflexologists believe that these points correspond to zones in the body and that massaging these points can relieve stress and prevent or treat disease. Reflexology is a holistic therapy that aims to restore and maintain the body's natural balance and encourage healing. Some reflexologists also believe that the health of a person can be assessed by feeling the points to detect imbalances or blockages in the flow of energy in the body. These blockages are felt as tenderness or a "crunchy" sensation.

Evidence shows that some early African tribes, the American Indians, early Egyptians, and the ancient Chinese knew about foot massage and reflexology. However, its revival was brought about by Dr. William Fitzgerald in the early 1920s. He found that he could anesthetize the ear by applying pressure to a certain part of the foot, and then perform minor ear operations. He went on to develop his theory that the body is divided into ten vertical zones running from the feet to the head and the hands, and that energy flows through these zones. He claimed that when the energy in the body is imbalanced, a crystalline deposit forms at the relevant reflex point on the foot. Massaging this to break it up frees the energy flow.

What happens at a reflexology session?

At your first appointment, the reflexologist will ask about your medical history before starting the treatment on your feet. Or, he or she may start the treatment on your hands if you have a health problem that affects your feet. During the treatment, which lasts between 30 minutes and 1 hour, you will either sit or lie down.

Reflexologists use their hands, and particularly their thumbs, to give the treatment. Gentle massage is used initially, followed by deep pressure. You may feel some brief discomfort or tenderness during the treatment. On the whole, the feelings you experience during a reflexology session should be relaxing and pleasant.

Does it work?

Nobody fully understands the way reflexology works, and there are no known connections in conventional medicine between organs or glands in the body and the reflex zones on the feet. Only a few scientific studies of reflexology have been undertaken, and a review of these studies found that, overall, reflexology has not been shown to be any more effective than placebo treatment. However, other studies have found that it could help alleviate premenstrual symptoms, reduce anxiety, help relieve symptoms of multiple sclerosis, and benefit people with diabetes.

Is it safe?

The safety of reflexology has not been the subject of rigorous scientific study. Reflexology can result in brief, mild pain during the treatment itself. People have reported feeling sick, sleepy, or tearful after a session. Some reflexologists believe that after a treatment people may experience a healing crisis, a cold feel, a cough, a skin rash, or a desire to go to the lavatory more often than usual. If you are pregnant or have a heart problem, thrombosis, a thyroid disorder, diabetes, or shingles, consult your doctor to see if reflexology is suitable for you. Professional reflexology associations insist that their members do not claim to be able to diagnose disease, because there have been reports of reflexologists making incorrect diagnoses.

A reflexology map of the feet that shows the zones of the body.

yoga

Yoga is a philosophy, a science, and an art, as well as a therapy. The word *yoga*, meaning "union" (with the soul) is, in the East, a way of working toward spiritual enlightenment. However, yoga does not need to be an all-consuming spiritual practice. In the West, it is more often practiced as a way of improving one's physical and mental well-being. It improves flexibility and strength, and can relieve physical ailments. It can also sharpen the intellect, improve concentration, calm the mind, and bring inner peace.

Where does yoga come from?

Yoga originated in India several thousand years ago. However, the philosophy of yoga was first ordered and written down about 2,000 years ago by the sage Patanjali. His work is known as the Yoga Sutra and it is still considered to be the most authoritative writing on yoga. There are eight limbs, or parts, to yoga, which together affect every aspect of life:

• Yama, or universal ethics for right living

• Niyama, or personal discipline

• Asanas, or the yoga postures

• Pranayama, or yoga breathing

• Pratyahara, or withdrawing the senses from the external world

• Dharana, or the concentration of the mind

• Dhyana, or meditation

• Samadhi, or enlightenment or the state of bliss and "truth."

In the West, yoga is usually taken to mean the practice of yoga postures, yoga breathing, and meditation.

Does it work?

Practiced regularly, in the recommended way, the yoga postures stretch and tone nearly every muscle and tendon in the body and move nearly all the joints through their complete range of movement. There is no doubt that this leads to an increase in suppleness and strength.

Yoga also has an effect on the internal organs of the body. For example, doing a headstand improves blood flow to the brain, and doing twists gently massages the digestive system and liver and can help eliminate toxins and waste. It is important to practice a complete range of postures to get the full benefit. These include standing postures, forward bends, back bends, neutral-type postures, twists, and inverted postures.

Whatever your ability at yoga, there are postures in each group that you can do. The breathing techniques of yoga are also beneficial, inducing relaxation, improving lung capacity, and increasing energy.

A substantial amount of scientific research into the benefits of yoga and studies have shown that yoga can help for a wide variety of health problems. For example, for people with back problems, it has been shown to help prevent further trouble, and it has also been found to help people with rheumatoid arthritis. Yoga breathing has been shown to reduce the frequency of asthma attacks and yoga meditation to benefit the heart and improve circulation.

Is it safe?

Essentially, yoga is safe and can be practiced by young and old alike, whatever their level of fitness, but the postures need to be practiced correctly, in the recommended sequence. Forcing your body into an advanced position that it is not ready for could lead to injury. It is important to remember that yoga is not a competition to see who can contort themselves into the most extreme position. Don't worry if you are not able to do a particular posture or hold it as long as someone else in a class. After all, yoga is for you, and if you practice regularly, you will be surprised how quickly your flexibility and strength improve.

People with certain diseases or injuries should take care with some postures and initially have careful supervision. If you are concerned that yoga might be risky for you, talk to your doctor or a qualified yoga teacher. Pregnant women also need to avoid certain postures at different times during their pregnancy. In fact, if you are pregnant and just starting to practice yoga, it is probably best to go to a special prenatal yoga class.

The different types of yoga

Yoga has become increasingly popular over the last few years, and classes are now available everywhere. How do you know which of the several different types of yoga is right for you? The following brief descriptions of the most common types can guide you to the type that might suit you. It is often best to try a class out, because whether you like the teacher is also important. There are different levels of yoga class, usually beginner, general, and intermediate. If you have not done yoga before, then a beginner class will be best, especially if you are stiff or unfit. An intermediate class is usually only for people who have been practicing for some years, because a good level of knowledge of the postures will be expected. A yoga session usually lasts from 1 to 2 hours, depending on the type of yoga and level of the class.

If you are just starting yoga, joining a class means that you get the correct instruction for the poses. The teacher will ensure that you don't strain yourself.

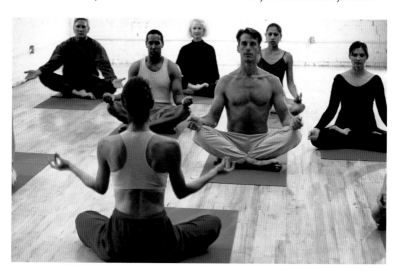

Hatha yoga is concerned with the correct use of the complete body. Today, it is the generic name given to the practice of yoga postures, breathing, and relaxation. It is probably the name you are most likely to come across. Many of the other of types of yoga are forms of hatha yoga.

Iyengar yoga was developed by B.K.S. Iyengar, who still teaches at his Institute in Puna, India. A synthesis of hatha and raja yoga (meditation), Iyengar yoga is now practiced all over the world. B.K.S. Iyengar systematically studied more than 200 yoga postures and breathing techniques and looked at how they relate to the anatomy of the body. From this he discovered that to get the best out of the postures and breathing, every part of the body must be positioned correctly.

Iyengar yoga, therefore, is characterized by precision and attention to detail, in order to get the correct alignment in the yoga postures. Although this type of yoga is physically demanding, various props (such as blocks, chairs, belts, and ropes) are commonly used to enable everyone, regardless of ability, age, or health status, to practice Iyengar yoga.

The use of props also makes Iyengar yoga a good type of yoga to practice if you are ill or injured in any way, preferably under the guidance of an experienced Iyengar yoga teacher to begin with.

Astanga vinyasa yoga, sometimes also called "Power yoga," was developed by Pattabhi Jois, who learned yoga from the same teacher as B.K.S. Iyengar. The postures practiced are similar to those used in Iyengar yoga, but are carried out in set series. Usually, the postures are performed quickly, one after the other, often connected by jumps, with an emphasis on controlling breathing.

This type of yoga encourages a buildup of heat in the body. Less emphasis is placed on the alignment of the body than in Iyengar yoga. It is a physically demanding system of yoga, and you should be relatively fit before attempting it.

Sivananda yoga is another form of hatha yoga, named after the great twentieth-century Indian yoga practitioner Swami Sivananda. It involves a specific set of breathing practices and postures, and is probably less physically taxing than Astanga or Iyengar yoga, at least in the beginning.

Yoga therapy is relatively new and is yoga specifically designed for people with a health problem. Yoga therapists are yoga teachers who have had additional training in how to use yoga to treat specific ailments. Yoga routines based on the yoga postures are practiced, but postures are included that might specifically benefit the problem, whereas those that might aggravate it are avoided.

Kundalini yoga involves specific practices to raise up through the spine the Kundalini energy that is said to reside at the base of the spine, and to bring health, harmony, and vitality when it is flowing well.

Tantric yoga is based on the belief that we can use the power of our senses and desires to transform and harmonize ourselves. It is the antithesis of the idea that we need to isolate ourselves from the world to reach enlightenment. It has also become a term that has come to mean sexual yoga, in which sexual intercourse is used to transform and increase energy.

Salute the sun

Practicing the yoga postures (asanas) is not just a type of physical exercise, because it involves the mind as well as the body. It is like a moving meditation, because as your mind concentrates on what your body is doing, it becomes focused and calm. You will notice the benefits from doing about 20–30 minutes of yoga regularly at home.

Try practicing the following sequence called "salute the sun," so called because it was traditionally practiced every day facing the rising and setting sun. It is reputed to increase flexibility and strength, and to relax and focus the mind. Begin by doing it about three times each day and building up to ten times. Remember to keep breathing as you do it.

1. Begin by standing up straight with your feet and inner ankles together and arms stretching down at your sides (tadasana, or mountain pose).

2. With a breath in, bring your arms straight up over your head, palms facing each other (urdhva hastasana).

3. Breathe out and bend forward at the hips, keeping your legs straight. The full posture is with your hands on the floor, but just go down as far as you can, and hold your legs where you feel comfortable (uttanasana).

4. Keeping your hands where they are, breathe in and straighten your back, trying to look up (uttanasana head up).

5. Bend your knees until your hands are flat on the floor and shoulderwidth apart. Then, breathe out and jump (or step if you have a knee or lower back problem) your feet back about 3 feet (1 meter) and a hipwidth apart so that your arms and legs are straight and you are making an upside-down **V** shape with your buttocks pointing at the ceiling. Keep your neck and head relaxed, and your hands and feet facing forward. Eventually, your feet should be flat on the floor. Take three breaths in this position (adho mukha svanasana, or downward facing dog).

6. Breath in and lower your hips toward the floor but a few inches above it, bringing your head and body forward through your arms. Push the floor away with your arms and stretch your spine up to the ceiling but look forward. Keep your legs straight and parallel to, but not touching, the floor. Roll your shoulders down and back. When you are able to, you can also roll from your toes onto the top of your feet (urdhva mukha svanasana, or upward facing dog).

7. Breath out and push your hips back up toward the ceiling so that you are in downward facing dog again (as in step 5). If you have rolled on to the tops of your feet, flip back onto your toes.

8. Breathe in and jump (or step) your foot forward to your hands so that you are in uttanasana head up (as in step 4).

9. Breath out and let your head hang down so that you are in uttanasana again (as in step 3).

10. Breath in and come up to urdhva hastasana (as in step 2).

11. Breath out and let your arms come down so that you are in tadasana again (as in step 1). Take two breaths in this posture, then start the sequence again.

When you have finished, lie down for a few minutes to relax. Lie flat on the floor with your legs together and straight, and a blanket under your head and neck for support. Let your arms fall out, palms upward, about 2 feet (0.5 meter) away from your body. Let your legs fall slightly apart, and close your eyes.

Tips for practicing yoga

- Practice on an empty stomach.
- Always wear unrestrictive clothing.
- Practice with bare feet.
- If your floor is slippery, get a nonslip mat.
- Keep the room warm.

aromatherapy

Aromatherapy is based on the use of concentrated essential oils extracted from plants to relieve symptoms of ill health and to aid good health. It is often used together with massage. Many toiletries contain essential oils.

What are essential oils?

Essential oils are not actually oils, but instead aromatic (fragrant) volatile essences, made up mainly of chemicals known as terpenes. They can be collected from a wide range of medicinal and culinary plants and are usually obtained by steam distillation. They are found in the flowers, leaves, roots, grasses, peels, resin, and barks of plants. Essential oils are absorbed through the skin and start to work within about 20 minutes. Only the volatile, aromatic parts of a plant are contained in essential oils, so the oils do not have the wide range of actions that herbal medicines that contain the whole plant do.

How are essential oils used?

Aromatherapists use essential oils in many ways, such as during a massage (see p.104) or as an inhalation, and you can put a few drops of an oil in your bathwater. Several hundred essential oils exist, and each is thought to have different healing properties. At your first aromatherapy consultation, the therapist will probably take a detailed medical history and ask questions about your diet, your lifestyle, and any health problems. From the information, the therapist will decide which oils are suitable. Sometimes one oil is used; other times a blend of two or three may be necessary. The therapist will massage you using the oils in a carrier oil.

Does aromatherapy work?

Aromatherapy is said to help relieve stress and to treat muscular aches and pains, asthma, eczema, digestive problems, menstrual and menopausal problems, headaches, and insomnia. However, most evidence supporting the use of aromatherapy is anecdotal, although a few clinical trials have assessed its effects. Research suggests that it can help to treat anxiety and improve well-being; however, it is possible to predict the effects of certain essential oils from their chemical makeup.

Is it safe?

Essential oils are concentrated and can be quite toxic, so care is needed. They are diluted in a vegetable oil, such as almond oil or grapeseed oil. Never take them internally or use them undiluted on the skin. Check with a professional therapist or your doctor before using an essential oil if you are pregnant or breast-feeding. Several essential oils should not be used during pregnancy, and some may get into breast milk. Orange, lemon, and bergamot essential oils can cause your skin to burn easily because they react with ultraviolet light, and many oils can aggravate skin conditions (such as fennel, rosemary, verbena, and lemongrass). Sage, anise, and hyssop oils may be toxic, and other oils should not be used by people with epilepsy (fennel and wormwood) or high blood pressure (rosemary and thyme). Some homeopaths advise against using the oils while taking a homeopathic remedy (see homeopathy p.126) because they believe that the strong aroma can prevent them from working.

Using essential oils at home

Health food shops, pharmacies, and herbal shops sell essential oils. Lavender, chamomile, tea tree, clary sage, geranium, sandalwood, and ylang-ylang oils are suitable oils to use at home. Although expensive, buying the pure oil is your best choice because cheaper oils may be diluted. Store, sealed, in a cool, dark place, out of the reach of children.

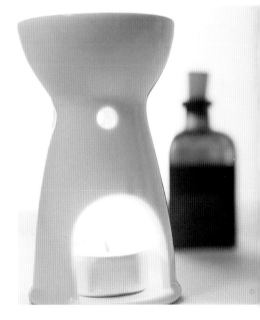

Many essential oils are ideal for use at home, perhaps in an oil burner.

herbal
medicine

Herbalism is probably the oldest therapy known to mankind. Today, most people in the world still use herbal remedies to treat disease, rather than expensive modern drugs. Even in the industrialized world, most pharmacies mainly sold herbs until the early twentieth century, and many modern medicines are derived from plants, the best known probably being aspirin from willow, digoxin from foxglove, and morphine from poppies. Scientific research is confirming many beliefs about the healing qualities of plants.

Minor illnesses have traditionally been self-treated within the home, whereas major illnesses have always been the domain of specially trained herbalists or healers. Like many complementary therapies, herbal medicine is often used to help the body cure itself, not just with relieving symptoms. Herbal practitioners believe that the delicate chemical balance of the whole herb is needed and do not isolate an active ingredient from a plant in the way that pharmaceutical companies do when making conventional drugs. Others believe that the active ingredients in a plant should be standardized to contain certain levels and thereby ensure potency. Remedies prescribed by a qualified herbalist may contain several herbs and are typically tailored to the individual patient. Such remedies can be made into various formulations, such as extracts, syrups, tinctures, lotions, inhalations, gargles, and washes. Today most people treating themselves rarely make their own remedy, because many ready-made herbal products (such as tablets, capsules, ointments, and creams) are available from health food shops and pharmacies. Keep in mind that you may need to take an herbal remedy for 2 to 3 months before noticing a difference in your condition.

Warning: Never take an herbal remedy with another medicine (prescribed or bought over-the-counter) without first consulting your doctor, pharmacist, or qualified herbalist to find out about any potentially dangerous drug-herb interactions.

Western herbalism

Many popular Western herbs are reputed to benefit us as we age or help with illnesses associated with aging. In the West, sage has traditionally been associated with longevity and wisdom (hence its name). It also contains estrogen-like substances that may help to prevent loss of calcium from bones and so reduce the risk of osteoporosis. Garlic is a useful herb to take as you get older; research suggests that it may help to reduce blood pressue, cholesterol levels and lower your risk of heart disease. Black cohosh has been scientifically shown to help with menopausal symptoms, and studies confirm the benefits of devil's claw for joint pain. Bladderwrack, or seaweed, is a good source of iodine and gently stimulates metabolism; it may be particularly useful for an underactive thyroid gland. Clinical trials have shown St. John's wort to be as effective as the antidepressant drug fluoxetine (Prozac) in treating mild to moderate depression, and it can be useful for women suffering emotional upsets during menopause. The leaf of the stinging nettle is an excellent source of vitamins and minerals and makes a useful tonic; it is also helpful for rheumatic disorders (see p.34) hay fever, and prostate problems (see p.40).

Ayurvedic medicine

Ayurvedic medicine is the traditional medicine of India and dates back to the Vedas, which were written in 2000 B.C. Ayurveda covers all aspects of health and disease, and takes into account physical, emotional, and spiritual well-being. It is concerned with the state of three vital energies, or doshas—vata, which is made up of the elements air and ether; pitta, which is fire and water; and kapha, which is water and earth. Herbal medicine forms just one part of the Ayurvedic system and is used along with yoga, massage, diet, and meditation, to balance the doshas and increase prana, or life energy. Gotu kola is probably one of the most well known Ayurvedic herbs in the West. It is a nerve tonic that is said to help induce mental calm and clarity; increase intelligence, memory, and longevity; and promote healing. Scientific trials have shown that frankincense, an herb commonly used in

Ayurvedic medicine, can help treat rheumatoid arthritis and, along with winter cherry, turmeric, and minerals, can help treat osteoarthritis. Frankincense and myrrh can both reputedly reverse the aging process. Winter cherry in Ayurvedic medicine is the equivalent of ginseng in Chinese medicine: It is said to be a powerful rejuvenating herb.

Chinese herbal medicine

Chinese herbal medicine works on the same principles as acupuncture (see p.100), and herbs are used to boost or disperse energy (qi) or to tone yin or yang using the same principles of TCM as acupuncture. Chinese herbalists rarely prescribe just one herb. Usually, a complex prescription of about 10 herbs is used. One of the most well-known Chinese herbs is ginseng (*Panax ginseng*). The Chinese have used the root of ginseng as a tonic for over 5,000 years, and its use has been widespread in the West for about 2,000 years. It is popular with elderly Chinese people for boosting energy and for treating chronic lung problems. However, scientific evidence for its benefits is limited and it should not be taken in high doses. If you take it regularly, have a short break every couple of months and limit the amount of caffeine and other stimulant herbs you consume at the same time. American ginseng tones yin more than the Chinese type and may be better for the very old, because they tend to be more yin deficient, or dry. Another important Chinese tonic herb is he shou wu (fo-ti), which is the dried root of *Polygonum multiforum*. Taoists believed that this herb may help to bring longevity, and it is also reputed to be effective with hair that is graying or falling out. It can be a particularly helpful tonic during menopause.

Native American herbs

The American plant ginkgo biloba encourages blood flow to the brain and appears to boost memory and reduce confusion in older people. The results of scientific research are promising, showing that it may be useful in treating circulatory problems and dementia. Native Americans originally used echinacea for snakebites, fevers, and wounds. Today, it is famous for its abilities to boost the immune system and has been the subject of much scientific research as a treatment for the common cold. Many people advocate taking it as a preventive measure for a week or two, particularly in the winter, if exposed to a cold, flu, or other infection.

Making a standard infusion

An infusion is made in a similar way to tea, using fresh or dried herbs. Follow these instructions to make three doses, which will last for 1 day:

1. Warm a teapot with hot water.
2. Put $3/4$ oz (25 g) of dried herbs or $2^1/_2$ oz (75 g) of fresh herbs in the empty pot.
3. Pour in 17 oz (500 ml) of freshly boiled water, and put the lid on the pot.
4. Leave to infuse for 10 minutes, then strain.
5. Add 1 teaspoon of honey to sweeten. Store any unused tea in a cool place.

Ginger

Ginger is one of the oldest and most universally used herbs in the world. It is used by each tradition—Western, Ayurvedic, and Chinese—in the same way. It is a warming herb, and is used for a range of problems, such as chills, colds, and poor circulation. It is also used to reduce nausea caused by travel sickness or during pregnancy, for example, and to treat digestive system problems such as indigestion, bloating, and flatulence. Both the root and the essential oil are used. Ginger's anti-inflammatory properties may help relieve the symptoms of osteoarthritis.

Native Americans first used echinacea to treat wounds and fevers. Now it is used to boost the immune system and to prevent colds.

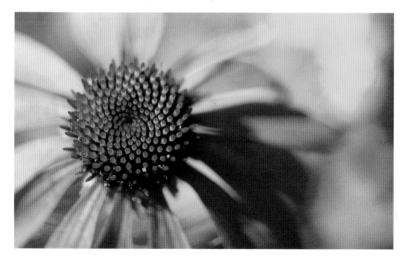

homeopathy

Homeopathy uses dilute preparations (remedies) made from animal, mineral, and plant sources to treat illness. Homeopaths believe that these remedies stimulate our bodies' own defenses and healing powers, known as the "vital force." Many also claim they are holistic, taking into account the person's mind, body, and spirit, rather than just treating the symptoms of a disease.

What is homeopathy?

Nobody is sure how homeopathy works, but it is based on the principle that "like cures like." Put simply, if a healthy person takes a poison and it causes a certain symptom, then the diluted poison is said to be a cure for that symptom. For example, the poisonous plant deadly nightshade, or belladonna, causes a throbbing headache, high fever, bright red face, palpitations, and hot, dry skin. Therefore, the homeopathic remedy belladonna is given to people who are feverish and have a sudden throbbing headache.

Samuel Hahnemann, the doctor who developed homeopathy in the eighteenth century, initially discovered that small amounts of cinchona bark, the treatment for malaria at the time, caused malaria-type fevers when he took it while healthy. Disillusioned with many of the dubious or dangerous medical treatments of the day, like blood-letting and the use of poisons such as arsenic and mercury, he went on to test many more substances on other healthy people, carefully noting the symptoms they caused and could therefore cure. He then developed a method of making homeopathic remedies from these substances by diluting and shaking them in water over and over again.

The resulting remedy may not even have one molecule of the original substance in it, but instead of weakening the substance, as one would expect, homeopaths claim that the more dilute a remedy is, the more effective it is.

What can homeopathy treat?

Homeopathy is used to treat almost any condition, except for mechanical problems such as a bad back, dislocation of a joint, or severe physical injury. Life-threatening events such as a heart attack, epileptic seizure, or asthma attack should not be treated with homeopathy alone, although some homeopathic remedies may be suitable for use with conventional medicines. Trained homeopaths are consulted for many chronic conditions, such as arthritis, eczema, menstrual problems, menopausal symptoms, and allergies. In addition, many people self-treat minor ailments with homeopathic remedies bought from their local health food shop or pharmacy (see box on p.128). However, it is not possible to reliably say which ailments are best treated with homeopathy. Studies of homeopathy have tended to focus on establishing whether or not the remedies are more effective than placebo. Although results of these studies have been inconsistent, when combined, they strongly suggest that homeopathy is more effective than placebo. However, more research is needed before it is possible to say which conditions homeopathic remedies can definitely help. Little evidence exists for or against using homeopathy for complicated or chronic problems.

Homeopathy and aging

The homeopathic remedy lycopodium is believed to help with hair loss and graying hair resulting from premature aging.

Is it safe?

Generally, homeopathy seems to be safe because the active ingredients of homeopathic remedies are present in such low concentrations. Many homeopaths claim that people can have a "healing" reaction to homeopathic remedies, during which their symptoms get worse before getting better. Such a reaction should be short-lived and is thought to be a necessary part of the healing process.

What happens at a homeopathic session?

A homeopathic consultation generally takes from between 45 minutes to 2 hours, during which time the practitioner asks detailed questions about your medical history, health, likes and dislikes, and emotional and mental states. Many homeopaths claim to treat each patient as an individual, attempting to identify the ideal remedy for that person's general constitution. This therapy style is known as classical homeopathy.

Some homeopaths prescribe a combination of remedies, a practice known as complex homeopathy. There are also homeopaths who prescribe on the basis of a conventional medical diagnosis or symptoms only. Once a remedy is prescribed, you should take it at least 30 minutes after a meal and should not eat or drink

SELF-HELP HOMEOPATHY

A limited range of low-potency homeopathic remedies is widely available in many pharmacies and health food shops for self-treatment. More and more people keep remedies at home for first-aid purposes and to treat minor ailments such as colds, headaches, and stress. For self-treatment, use 6C or 12C potency remedies. The following remedies are useful to keep in the first-aid cabinet:

Remedy	Formulation	Main Use
• Arnica	Tablets	Shock or injury
	Ointment (unbroken skin)	Bruising or swelling
• Apis	Tablets	Stings, inflammation, or burning pains
• Carbo veg	Tablets	Digestive problems
• Hypericum	Tincture	Cuts and grazes
• Ruta	Tablets or ointment	Strains and sprains
• Urtica	Tablets	Burns

Warning: Always consult a professional homeopath for a chronic or serious problem.

anything for at least 10 minutes afterward. Some homeopaths will warn you against using any strong-tasting or stong-smelling substances (including toothpaste, peppermint, alcohol, spicy foods, or essential oils) because they believe these can cancel out the effects of a homeopathic remedy.

If your condition is acute, you may only need to take one dose of a remedy to see an improvement. Chronic conditions may need to be treated for many months, and you may need to consult your homeopath on several occasions and take more than one remedy before getting better.

Homeopathy for hot flashes

Menopausal symptoms, such as hot flashes, are not a serious threat to your health, but for some women they can be debilitating and upsetting. At least three homeopathic remedies may be worth trying and are safe alternatives to treatments such as hormone replacement therapy. Belladonna can help relieve hot flashes that affect the head and face, sepia is useful for hot flashes that occur at the same time as anxiety attacks, and pulsatilla is good for hot flashes or a sweaty face.

Tissue salts

Tissue salts are a type of homeopathic remedy made from minerals like quartz. They are often used by homeopaths, but they can also be bought over-the-counter and used for self-treatment. Tissue salts are mainly used for minor ailments such as coughs, colds and sore throats, hay fever, indigestion, nonserious skin conditions, headaches, stress, and muscle pains.

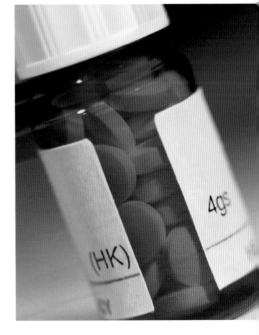

Homeopathic remedies come as tablets, pills, granules, powders, and tinctures.

naturopathy
and hydrotherapy

Developed in the nineteenth century, naturopathy is a
complete system of treating ill health that is based on the
premise that, in the right conditions, our bodies cure
themselves by innate vital forces.

Naturopathy

Naturopaths believe that lifestyle managment centered in diet, exercise, stress reduction,
adequate sleep, and detoxification enable the body to restore good health and
promote longevity. Naturopaths are often trained in other disciplines, such as
osteopathy (see p.108) acupuncture (see p.100), and homeopathy (see p.126)
Naturopathic schools are licensed by several states.

The concept of homeostasis

An underlying principle of naturopathy is that our bodies are naturally self-regulating.
This is known as homeostasis, which is a state of healthy biochemical balance.
Disease is the result of an unhealthy lifestyle and diet that undermines the body's
natural self-regulating mechanisms and leads to illness. Naturopaths believe that such
signs and symptoms as inflammation, fever, and pain are indications that the body
is working toward harmony and that it is not always a good idea to surpress them
with drugs. They believe that these symptoms reflect the body's way of healing and
that they are not necessarily bad for you just because they are unpleasant.
Naturopathic treatments aim to restore the body to a healthy balance—a healthy
homeostasis.

The naturopathic session

Diagnosing what is wrong and why homeostasis has broken down is an important part
of naturopathic treatment. On your first visit to a naturopath, you will be questioned

about your medical history, family history, lifestyle, and symptoms. Usually, you will have your blood and urine analyzed to assess glucose, vitamin, and mineral levels, and sometimes a sample of your hair will be sent away for analysis or you may be referred for X rays. The naturopath will give you a physical examination, looking at your eyes, skin, nails, mouth, and tongue; listening to your heart and lungs with a stethoscope, and take your blood pressure. The naturopath will use all the information to assess how you are functioning and what your vital forces are like, as well as to diagnose what is wrong with you physically.

Essentially, the treatment that will be recommended will either be mainly anabolic (building up), if you are nutritionally deficient and have had your symptoms for some time, or catabolic (breaking down), if the problem seems to be due to buildup of toxins. Naturopathic treatment is as natural as possible. Measures to build you up might include rest and relaxation, massage and gentle manipulation, a whole-food diet, and vitamin and mineral supplements. Measures to break down toxins may include elimination diets, fasting, hydrotherapy and colonic irrigation (see p.133), and exercise and manipulation.

Naturopaths recognize that poor body posture, misalignment of joints, and muscle spasms all affect health. Many are trained in manipulative techniques (see osteopathy and chiropractic, p.108), or they may recommend that you start practicing the Alexander technique (see p.74) or yoga (see p.114) to realign your body. They often use herbal (see p.122) and/or homeopathic remedies (see p.126).

The role of emotions in ill health is considered very important and they often spend time counseling patients, and teaching relaxation techniques (see p.82).

Dietary measures

Naturopaths basically recommend a similar diet to that outlined in the section on nutrition and healthy eating (see p.54)—that is, one high in fiber and low in saturated fats, with lots of fresh fruit and vegetables. Preferably, the foods should be organically grown and contain no chemical additives or preservatives. The naturopath might simply recommend increasing the amount of vitamin- and mineral-rich foods you eat. Or, he or she might recommend going on an elimination diet to identify the foods you are allergic to or intolerant of, or fasting to detoxify your body.

Fasting

Under the right conditions, a fast can be beneficial and can help to restore good health. It should not be confused with starvation. A fast can give the body a rest and let it divert energy to removing toxins and restoring harmony, rather than digesting and storing food. A fast does not have to mean not eating anything. It can involve eating only one food or one group of foods exclusively for a set amount of time. One of the most well known single-food diets is the grape cure. However, it is inadvisable to fast without being supervised by a qualified practitioner.

Evidence for naturopathy

Conventional medical experts now accept many of the beliefs of naturopathy and a wealth of evidence now supports them. For example, no one would question the benefits of the whole-food diet that it advocates, that pesticides and chemical additives can be harmful to our health, or that we should restrict the amount of saturated animal fats we eat. Many naturopathic beliefs about vitamins and minerals have been backed up by scientific research, although conventional medicine generally still does not support using megadoses.

As far as the nondietary naturopathic beliefs are concerned, it is universally recognized that a lack of exercise and too much stress can lead to ill health. However, many conventional medical experts question the naturopathic diagnosis of candida (thrush) in the gut as a common cause of symptoms, and the value of colonic irrigation (see p.133) has yet to be scientifically studied.

Naturopathic principles could be used to help in any illness, and are gaining rapid acceptance by the general public and by the mainstream of medicine.

Hydrotherapy

Water has been used as a therapy for thousands of years. Today, hydrotherapy uses water inside and outside the body to prevent illness, boost vital energy, improve circulation, and restore and cleanse the body. Both hot and cold water are used, as well as steam and ice, baths, saunas, hot and cold compresses and wraps, whirlpools, and water jets.

Seawater treatment (thalassotherapy) is also said to be healing. Hydrotherapy is mainly used for arthritic problems, back pain, sports injuries, respiratory conditions,

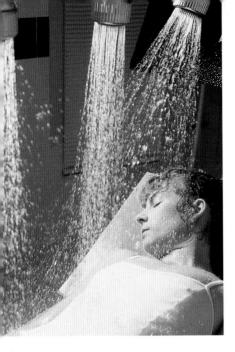

Taking a cold shower is a hydrotherapy technique to boost the immune system.

poor circulation, menstrual problems, stress, headaches, and chronic tiredness. Not only is hydrotherapy widely used by naturopaths, it is also an integral part of conventional medicine, where it is mainly used by physiotherapists.

Boosting your immune system

Hydrotherapy techniques can be used to boost your immune system and prevent and treat colds and other illnesses. One way of doing this is to warm yourself up in a hot bath or steam room; briskly rub yourself down with a cold, wet cloth; then wrap yourself in a towel. Alternatively, take a cold shower every morning. Scientific research shows that doing this for 6 months or more can reduce the frequency and severity of colds.

Irrigating the colon

Colonic irrigation is a detoxification technique also called colonic hydrotherapy. Therapists claim that the walls of the colon (large intestine) can have fecal material stuck to them, which can be reabsorbed into the bloodstream, causing symptoms of ill health such as chronic tiredness, digestive problems, skin disorders, and headaches. Colonic irrigation aims to get rid of this material by flushing it out with water. The water, which is filtered and may contain vitamins, minerals, or homeopathic remedies, is administered into the colon through a tube inserted into the rectum. The patient, who lies down during the procedure, holds the water in the colon for a couple of minutes each time.

Colonic irrigation can be repeated several times at each session, which last for around 45 minutes. A course of treatment usually consists of about six sessions.

conventional
medicine

Conventional medicine has literally hundreds of drugs available to treat human diseases; no drug is yet available to stop or even slow the aging process. However, certain drugs have been shown to increase life expectancy in specific groups of people—for example, those who have had a heart attack or who have cancer or heart failure. Other drugs are also being used experimentally to see if they can slow the general signs of aging. It is the latter that we will concentrate on.

Conventional medicine also uses surgery to treat disease and to try and reverse some of the effects of aging, and some experimental techniques might even increase the human life span in the near future. Conventional medicine also promotes disease prevention through a healthy diet and lifestyle, vaccination programs, disease screenings, and drug therapy. This includes drugs to lower high blood pressure and so prevent heart attacks and strokes, and the anticancer drug tamoxifen (Nolvadex) to prevent certain types of breast cancer.

Using hormones to beat aging

Several hormones have been implicated in the aging process, because the levels of many hormones change as we grow older. The most obvious are the female sex hormones, estrogen and progesterone, synthetic combinations of which many women take during menopause as hormone replacement therapy (see menopause on p.38). However, several other hormonal products are advocated as antiaging drugs—but do they work and how safe are they?

DHEA The full name for this hormone is dehydroepiandrosterone. It is produced by the adrenal glands and is the most abundant steroid hormone in our bodies. It is used to make the sex hormones testosterone, estrogen, and progesterone. Proponents of DHEA believe that it may be able to boost the immune system and protect against infection; reduce the risk of heart disease, osteoporosis, and cancer; prevent the onset of type 2 diabetes; help with memory loss; and lengthen life expectancy. However, not enough good research has been done, and no studies have looked at its long-term effects. Although it is possible to buy DHEA capsules, DHEA is not an FDA-approved drug, and so cannot be marketed for medical purposes. DHEA may aggravate certain cancers, and adverse effects include the growth of facial hair and deepening of the voice in women, and acne in men.

Human growth hormone This hormone is made by the pituitary gland and stimulates growth and repair in the body. The claimed benefits for this drug seem impressive. Advocates of human growth hormone believe it can make your skin less wrinkled and thicker, your bones stronger, and your muscle mass increase. It is also purported to result in weight loss without dieting, a stronger immune system, better sleep, a higher energy level, improved sexual performance, better exercise performance, lower blood pressure and cholesterol levels, better eyesight, improved memory, and the regrowth of and improved functioning of many organs. Yet this hormone is available only with a doctor's prescription, and is only used to treat adults and children with proven deficiencies in human growth hormone. This is because there is no conclusive evidence to support its alleged health benefits, and because it can have serious side effects, ranging from severe headaches and visual problems to brain swelling and joint problems. However, it is claimed that adverse effects are rare if a low dosage is given. What's more, DHEA is very expensive.

Melatonin This hormone is produced by the pineal gland, a tiny gland in the middle of the brain. It is thought to be responsible for our body clocks and small studies have shown that taking low doses of melatonin seems to help prevent jet lag and treat insomnia in the short term. However, some people claim that it can also extend life, keep us youthful, and combat a whole range of chronic diseases—and that it is also safe. Unfortunately, although some evidence shows that melatonin can extend the life span of mice by as much as 25 percent, no solid evidence from human studies supports these claims. In addition, we actually don't know whether it is safe or not, especially in the long term. Furthermore, the doses advocated in the consumer arena are far higher than levels of melatonin found in the body, and this could result in unforeseen adverse effects in the future.

Testosterone This male sex hormone is known to promote the buildup of muscle, skin, and bone. It is produced by the testicles and increases greatly in concentration during puberty. Levels of the hormone start to decline in middle age, which is purported to lead to loss of sex drive and impotence, tiredness, depression, painful joints, loss of muscle, osteoporosis, dry skin, and weight loss. The growing trend is to use testosterone to treat what has been dubbed the "andropause," or male menopause, although whether this condition actually exists is debatable. Considerable caution is needed with this hormone, because taking testosterone can result in dangerous adverse reactions if given to men with already normal levels, and it may stimulate the growth of preexisting prostate tumors and may reduce levels of protective high-density lipoprotein cholesterol levels in the body. Conventional medicine only uses testosterone in men who have been castrated or who have a recognized deficiency in the hormone, due to either pituitary or testicular disease.

Future antiaging medicines

Antiaging strategies are being investigated in the world of pharmaceuticals. The most exciting are either based on removing free radicals, such as synthetic catalytic scavengers (SCS), or blocking or mimicking the effects of the enzyme telomerase, which controls the "biological" clocks (known as telomeres) in all our cells, that control the rate of cell division. Other areas of active research include looking at chemicals that boost the link between brain cells to keep our brains functioning well, drugs to stimulate the growth of organs and blood vessels, and gene therapies to delay age-related hearing and sight problems.

Synthetic catalytic scavengers These compounds are still in the experimental stage, but it is thought that they could extend life span by "mopping up" free radicals. Free radicals are continuously being made in the body as part of its defense against bacteria, but they are also thought to cause damage and aging (see antioxidants, p.58). Our bodies produce antioxidants such as the enzyme super oxide dismutase (SOD), but normal levels may be inadequate in the polluted world we live in. Scientists have now discovered a group of compounds called synthetic catalytic scavengers (SCS), and the first drug in this group to be developed has been shown to increase the life span in the nematode worm. The manufacturer is now seeking permission to study the drug's effects in human patients who have had strokes or skin burns from radiotherapy. During these studies, the researchers will be looking for signs that the drug is slowing the aging process.

Telomerase-based drugs This research is not as far advanced as that for SCS, but if drugs could be developed that mimic telomerase, they could possibly extend the lives of ordinary cells and may even reverse the aging process. Conversely, drugs that block the effect of telomerase might be used to stop the spread of cancer cells.

Screening for cancer

Regular screening for some common cancers is recommended because cancer is more easily treated if caught early. Symptoms don't usually develop until there are millions of cancer cells or the primary cancer is about the size of a small grape.

Breast cancer Mammograms, ultrasound, thermography and genetic testing are all used to screen for cancer or an increased risk of cancer. If a mother or sister has had breast cancer, then it is advisable to start having annual mammograms at about age 40. Sometimes ultrasound is used for younger women, who naturally tend to have more lumpy breasts, for which mammograms are not suitable. Genetic testing is used to look for two genes—known as BRCA1 and BRCA2—that, if mutated, mean an increased risk of breast cancer. About 85 percent of women with a mutated BRCA1 gene will have breast cancer by the time they are age 70. Some debate still exists as to whether breast self-examination is beneficial.

Cervical cancer All women, regardless of age, should have a cervical, or Papanicolaou, smear every 3 years to check for precancerous or cancer cells.

Testicular cancer This is on the increase and is the most common cancer in men between ages 20 and 35. If caught early, 90 percent of cases are curable. Men should examine their testicles regularly, in a warm bath or shower, by rolling each testicle between thumb and finger. A healthy testicle should feel smooth, apart from the soft tube toward the back that carries and stores sperm. Any change in a testicle (such as a hard lump, change in size or firmness, or any pain or discomfort) should be examined by a doctor.

plastic

surgery

Plastic, or cosmetic, surgery is becoming more and more common. Many people who have plastic surgery do so to increase their confidence in their appearance, such as for a cleft lip, badly broken nose, or a large birthmark. However, plastic surgery is also on the increase to try and reverse the effects of aging, such as facial wrinkling, drooping eyelids, age spots, broken blood vessels, or sagging breasts and abdomen. Techniques include facelifts, chin tucks, removal of bags under the eyes, collagen implants, breast reduction, and liposuction (fat removal).

Facelifts

The first facelift was carried out over 100 years ago by a German surgeon. Now, thousands are carried out each year. Facelifts help to make a face look younger, but they are not a cure-all, and a person's lifestyle and diet before and after surgery can have a big impact on how successful the operation is and how long the effects last. Plastic surgery is more successful the thinner you are, but like all surgery, it can have complications such as pain and scarring, and the usual risks of general anesthesia. It is vital to pick the best plastic surgeon possible for your operation. Plastic surgery is an art, and a bad job can result in lasting disfigurement.

Chemosurgery

This procedure is sometimes advocated to remove fine lines on older skin. Superficial chemosurgery, or skin peeling, involves destroying the top layer (the epidermis) of the skin with a solution containing a caustic (burning) substance, such as resorcinol. The solution is removed after a specific length of time. Initially, the skin forms a crust, which falls off after about a week to reveal "new" pink skin. Deep peeling uses a combination of stronger chemicals, such as phenol, to remove part of the second layer of the skin (the dermis) as well. The chemicals are applied up to four times. These procedures are painful, and the results vary. Although chemosurgery can result in the skin looking younger and less wrinkled, the effects last only a few months, after which the skin looks as it did before. However, skin peeling can remove age spots, freckles, and superficial scars.

Dermabrasion is a procedure that involves removing the top layer of the skin using a high-speed motorized wire brush. It is carried out under general anesthesia and is supposed to result in a similar effect to chemosurgery, but it may be even less effective.

Hair transplants

Hair transplant methods are becoming more sophisticated, but many men are still dissatisfied with the results. Hair grafts can involve transplanting a single hair at a time (micrografts); very tiny plugs of hair-bearing skin with 2–6 hairs (microblend grafts); tiny plugs of skin with eight hairs (blend grafts); or plugs with about 100 hairs (plug grafts). At each operation, about 300 to 400 single hairs are transplanted, resulting in a thin covering of hair. To get thicker hair coverage, you need about 650 hairs in each square inch, and the procedure is only suitable for men who are just beginning to lose their hair or who want their hairline extended forward. Microblend grafts are suitable for similar problems but can result in slightly thicker hair coverage. Blend grafting is the most common procedure used and is suitable for men who are thinning all over. Scalp reduction may be performed to reduce the size of a bald patch.

Botox injections

Injections of botulinum A toxin (Botox) were marketed as a treatment of muscle spasm in the face and neck. They work by paralyzing the muscles they are injected into, which is how they also work to reduce wrinkles and sagging. The effects wear off after a few months, and the injections can have some adverse effects, such as paralysis of other distant muscles, rash, transient burning sensations at the site of injection, difficulty in swallowing, dry mouth, double or blurred vision, or headache.

useful organizations

Acupuncture
American Academy of Medical
Acupuncture
5820 Wilshire Blvd., Suite 500
Los Angeles, CA 90036
Telephone: (213) 937-5514
www.medicalacupuncture.org

Aging
Alliance for Aging Research
2021 K St. NW, Suite 305
Washington, DC 20006
Telephone: (202) 293-2856
www.agingresearch.org

American Association of Retired
Persons (AARP)
601 E St. NW
Washington, DC 20049
Telephone: (202) 434-2300
www.aarp.org

American Geriatric
Society/Foundation for Health in
Aging
The Empire State Building
305 Fifth Ave., Suite 801
New York, NY 10018
Telephone: (212) 755-6820
www.healthinaging.org

Alexander technique
North American Society of Teachers
of the Alexander Technique
3010 Hennepin Ave. S., Suite 10
Minneapolis, MN 55408
Telephone: (612) 824-5066
www.sportstherapy.com/alexan.htm

Aromatherapy
National Association for Holistic
Aromatherapy
4509 Interlake Ave, N., #233
Seattle, WA 98103-6773
Telephone: (206) 547-2164
www.naha.org

Chiropractic
American Chiropractic Association
1701 Clarendon Blvd.
Arlington, VA 22209
Telephone: (800) 986-4636
www.amerchiro.org

Diabetes
American Diabetes Association
ATTN: Customer Service,
1701 N. Beauregard St.
Alexandria, VA 22311
Telephone: (800) 342-2383
www.diabetes.org

Digestive Health
American Gastroenterological
Association (American Digestive
Health Foundation)
National Office
7910 Woodmont Ave., Suite 700
Bethesda, MD 20814
Telephone: (301) 654-2055
www.gastro.org

Heart Disease and Stroke
American Heart Association (AHA)
American Stroke Association (ASA)
National Center, 7272 Greenville Ave.
Dallas, TX 75231
Telephone (AHA): (800) 242-8721
Telephone (ASA): (888) 478-7653
www.americanheart.org
www.strokeassociation.org

Herbal medicine
American Herbalists Guild
P.O. Box 1683
Soquel, CA 95073
Telephone: (408) 464-2441
www.americanherbalistsguild.com

Homeopathy
National Centre for Homeopathy
801 N. Fairfax St., Suite 306
Alexandria, VA 22314
Telephone: (703) 548-7790
www.homeopathic.org

Insomnia
American Academy of Sleep
Medicine (formerly American Sleep
Disorders Association)
6301 Bandel Rd. NW, Suite 101
Rochester, MN 55901
Telephone: (507) 287-6006
www.aasmnet.org

Massage
American Massage Therapy
Association
820 Davis St., Suite 100
Evanston, IL 60201-4444
Telephone: (708) 864-0123
www.amtamassage.org

Memory Loss and Dementia
Alzheimer's Association
919 N. Michigan Ave., Suite 1100
Chicago, IL 60611-1676
Telephone: (800) 272-3900
www.alz.org

Menopause
American Menopause Foundation
National Headquarters,
350 Fifth Ave., Suite 2822
New York, NY 10118
Telephone: (212) 714-2398
www.americanmenopause.org

Naturopathy
American Association of
Naturopathic Physicians
P.O. Box 20386
Seattle, WA 98102
Telephone: (206) 323-7610
www.naturopathic.org

Nutrition
American Dietetic Association
216 W. Jackson Blvd.
Chicago, IL 60606-6995
Telephone: (312) 899-0040
www.eatright.org

**Orthopedic Medicine and
Prolotherapy**
American Association of Orthopedic
Medicine
30897 C.R. 356-3, P.O. Box 4997
Buena Vista, CO 81211
Telephone: (800) 992-2063
www.aaomed.org

Osteopathy
American Academy of Osteopathy
3500 DePauw Blvd., Suite 1080
Indianapolis, IN 46268-1136
Telephone: (317) 879-0563
www.academyofosteopathy.org

American Osteopathic Association
142 E. Ontario St.
Chicago, IL 60611
Telephone: (312) 280-5800
www.aoa-net.org

Osteoporosis
National Osteoporosis Foundation
1232 22nd St., NW
Washington, DC 20037-1292
Telephone: (202) 223-2226
www.nof.org

Physiotherapy
American Physical Therapy
Association
1111 North Fairfax St.
Alexandria, VA 22314-1488
Telephone: (703) 684-2782
www.apta.org

Prostate and Impotence
American Prostate Society
7188 Ridge Rd
Hanover, MD 21076
Telephone: (410) 859-3735
www.ameripros.org

American Urological Association
Headquarters Office
1120 N. Charles St.
Baltimore, MD 21201
Telephone: (410) 727-1100
www.auanet.org/patient

Reflexology
Reflexology Association of America
(RAA)
4012 S. Rainbow St., K-PMB #K585
Las Vegas, NV 89103-2059
Telephone: (978) 799-7955
www.reflexology-usa.org

Yoga
Yoga Journal
2054 University Ave., Suite 600
Berkeley, CA 94704
Telephone: (510) 841-9200
www.yogajournal.com

glossary

ACE inhibitors a group of drugs used to treat high blood pressure and heart failure, and after a heart attack.

Adrenaline (epinephrine) a hormone produced in the body by the adrenal glands, and also used as a drug to treat severe allergic reactions and during a heart attack.

Allergen a substance that triggers an allergic reaction in the body, such as pollen in people who have hay fever.

Alpha reductase inhibitors a group of drugs used to treat an enlarged prostate gland (benign prostatic hyperplasia).

Anaphylaxis also known as anaphylactic shock, is a life-threatening allergic reaction that comes on very quickly and needs immediate treatment. Symptoms include sudden itching, difficulty in breathing, swelling of the face, and very low blood pressure.

Anti-androgens a group of drugs that block the effects of male sex hormones and are used to treat prostate gland disorders.

Beta-blockers a group of drugs used to treat high blood pressure, heart failure, angina (chest pain due to heart disease), abnormal heart rhythms, and after a heart attack. They are also sometimes used to relieve symptoms of anxiety.

Bisphosphonates a group of drugs used to prevent bone loss and treat osteoporosis in postmenopausal women, as well as bone disorders such as Paget's disease and bone cancer.

Calcitonin a drug that helps to regulate bone turnover, so is used in the management of osteoporosis in postmenopausal women, as well as other bone disorders.

Calcium channel blockers a group of drugs used to treat high blood pressure, abnormal heart rhythms, and angina (chest pain due to heart disease).

Candida a fungal infection that can cause thrush.

Cartilage special tough tissue attached to bones, to protect them.

Cerebrospinal fluid the clear fluid that flows around the brain and in the spinal column.

Chronic fatigue syndrome also known as myalgic encephalitis or ME, this is a condition that some people are thought to develop after a viral infection, but its cause is unclear. It can last for months or even years and is characterized by symptoms such as extreme tiredness and aches and pains, headaches, memory loss, depression, and sleep problems.

Clonidine a drug used to treat high blood pressure, migraine, and flushing during menopause.

Clot busting drugs a group of drugs used immediately after a heart attack to break up any blood clots and prevent further damage.

Collagen a type of protein that helps make up the connective tissue in the body.

Congenital disorder a medical condition present at birth that has either been inherited or has developed in the womb.

Corticosteroids a group of drugs that reduce inflammation in the body and are used in the management of asthma, eczema, allergies, rheumatic diseases, and so forth. The adrenal glands in the body also produce natural corticosteroid.

Dermatologist a doctor who specializes in treating skin disorders.

Detoxification a process that involves eliminating toxins from the body, such as through fasting.

Diabetic neuropathy a condition that occurs in people with diabetes, in which the nerves in the hands and feet stop working properly.

Diuretics drugs that work by increasing urine production, which are used to treat high blood pressure and heart failure.

DNA the substance found in most living organisms that carries genetic information.

Enzyme substances (made by cells) that are needed to make certain biological processes take place.

Essential fatty acids (EFAs) a group of unsaturated fatty acids that are vital for normal growth and which we have to get from what we eat, because our bodies can't make them.

Glitazones a group of drugs used in the management of type 2 diabetes.

Gonadorelin analogues a group of drugs used in the treatment of cancer of the prostate, fibroids in the womb, and endometriosis.

Hormones substances produced by glands in the body that are vital for the normal functioning and growth of the body.

Hydrocortisone a hormone produced by the body, which is also available as a synthetic corticosteroid (see above) in medicines applied locally, such as to the skin, eyes or ears, to reduce inflammation.

Hysterectomy an operation to remove the womb (uterus), and sometimes the ovaries as well.

Mammogram a type of scan used to examine the breasts for lumps.

Metformin a drug used in the management of type 2 diabetes.

Methotrexate a drug used in the treatment of rheumatoid arthritis, psoriasis, and cancer.

Minoxidil a drug used in the management of high blood pressure and for baldness.

MUSE a special device containing alprostadil, a drug used to treat impotence, which is used to insert the drug directly into the urethra in the penis.

Neurotransmitters chemicals produced in the body at nerve endings that transmit nerve signals from one nerve to another or to muscles.

Noradrenaline a hormone produced in the body. It is also used as a drug when someone has acute low blood pressure or a cardiac arrest.

NSAIDs stands for nonsteroidal anti-inflammatory drugs, which are used to reduce inflammation and pain, for example due to injury, arthritis, menstrual pains, and so on.

Opiates a group of centrally acting painkillers, such as morphine and codeine.

Penicillamine a drug known as a disease-modifying drug (DMARD), used mainly in the treatment of rheumatoid arthritis.

Pilates an exercise technique that tones the muscles of the body to increase their flexibility and strength.

Pituitary gland a gland situated in the brain that secretes hormones that trigger other glands to secrete their hormones.

Raloxifene a drug used to prevent and treat osteoporosis in postmenopausal women.

Rickets a condition due to vitamin D deficiency, in which the bones soften and bend.

Scurvy a condition due to vitamin C deficiency, the symptoms of which include bleeding gums, loose teeth, a tendency to bruise easily, and swollen joints.

Selective alpha-blockers a group of drugs used to treat symptoms of benign prostatic hyperplasia (enlarged prostate gland).

Shingles a disease due to the herpes varicella zoster virus (the same virus that causes chickenpox), in which the virus travels along nerves to the skin, causing a lot of pain and a localized rash.

Sildenafil a drug used to treat impotence and widely known by its trade name Viagra.

Statins a group of drugs used to lower cholesterol levels in the blood.

Sulphonylureas a group of drugs used in the management of type 2 diabetes.

Taoism a philosophy that originated in China. The Tao is loosely translated as "the Way."

Thyroid gland a gland in the neck responsible for secreting several hormones including thyroxine, which acts on all the cells in the body to control the rate at which food is converted into energy.

Trichologists people who perform hair analysis.

Ultrasound a type of scan used, for example, to examine the fetus in the womb or to examine the breasts for lumps.

index

A
abdominal breathing 83–85
accidents 53
acetylcholinesterase inhibitors 45
acupressure 93, 103
acupuncture 21, 31, 35, 39, 43, 81, 93, 100–102
addiction 20
adrenaline 78
aerobic exercise 65, 66
aging 11–14
alcohol 20, 22, 80
Alexander technique 74, 75
alpha reductase inhibitor 41
Alzheimer's disease 44, 45
antidepressants 39
antioxidants 56–58
aromatherapy 81, 120, 121
arthritic conditions 34, 35
aspirin 25, 31
atherosclerosis 22
attitudes 52
autogenics 81, 86
Ayurvedic medicine 35, 39, 43, 107, 123, 124

B
back pain 30–33
back twists 32, 33
bad habits, stopping 20, 21
baldness 96, 97
Bate's method 47
biofeedback 81, 86, 87
bisphosphonates 37
blood pressure 19, 23, 24
body mass index (BMI) 53
Botox injections 139
breathing, abdominal 81, 83–85
bupropion 21
buserelin 41

C
caffeine 80
calcitonin 37
calcium 36, 57, 59, 62
cancer 56, 95, 137
chemosurgery 138–139
chilblains 25
Chinese medicine 35, 43, 45, 46, 89, 100, 103, 106, 124
chiropractic 31, 108–111
chitosan 27

cholesterol 23
chondroitin 35, 59
chromium 29, 62
chronic health conditions 8, 17, 19
circulatory diseases 22–27
clonidine 39
coenzyme Q10 59
cognitive-behavioral therapy 81
colds 17
colonic irrigation 133
complementary medicine 9, 16, 98–133
complex carbohydrates 54
conventional medicine 8, 134–137
cortisol 13
cosmetic surgery 138, 139
counseling 21, 39, 42, 81
cult groups 80
cycling 66, 72
cyproterone acetate 41

D
deafness 49
deep breathing 83–85
dehydroepiandrosterone 135
dementia 44
depression 52, 81
DHEA 135
diabetes 28, 29
diet 22, 23, 28, 45, 54, 55, 93, 131
disease 16
disease prevention 64, 65
disease modifying antirheumatic drug 35
doctors 8, 15, 16–19, 67
donepezil 45
drugs 21, 34, 35, 80, 137

E
ears 46–49
echinacea 41, 124
emergency treatment 18, 19
emotions 52
energy 99, 100, 103
Epsom salt bath 35
essential fatty acids (EFA) 44, 55, 59
essential oils 43, 93, 120
estrogen 13, 38, 93
exercise 22, 24, 31, 32, 37, 45, 64–67, 80

exercises 32, 33, 43, 66, 68–71, 94, 95
eyes 46–49

F
face exercises 94
facelifts 138
fasting 132
fats 23, 54
Feldenkrais method 75, 76
fiber 54, 56
finasteride 41
fish oils 35
fitness 65
Fitzgerald, William 112
food sensitivities 57
free radicals 13, 58
fruit 54, 56, 57
future medicines 136, 137

G
galantamine 45
garlic 29, 123
ginkgo biloba 43, 44, 45, 124
ginseng 43, 124
glaucoma 48
glitazone 29
glucosamine 35, 59
gonadorelin analogues 41
goserelin 41

H
Hahnemann, Samuel 126
hair transplants 139
hands, exercises 95
head massage 107
healing crisis 130
health 52, 53
heart 22–27, 38
Hellerwork 76
herbal medicine 39, 81, 90, 122–125
high-density lipoprotein (HDL) cholesterol 23
hobbies 80
holistic approach 98, 99
homeopathy 39, 126–129
homeostasis 130
hormone replacement therapy 37-39
hormones 13, 134–136
human growth hormone 13, 135
hydrocortisone 78

hydrotherapy 25, 133
hypertension 24
hypnosis 43
hypnotherapy 87

I

ibuprofen 31
immune system, boosting 132
impotence 42, 43
indoramin 41
infusions 125
injuries, sport 73
insulin 13, 29
integrated medicine 99
Iyengar, B.K.S. 117

J

jet lag 91
Jois, Pattabhie 117

L

life expectancy 9
life force 99, 100
life purpose 15
low-density lipoprotein (LDL)
    cholesterol 23
lycopodium 127

M

macular degeneration 47
magnesium sulphate 35
male menopause 136
massage 31, 45, 81, 93,
    104–107
McTimoney-Corley chiropractic
    111
medical checkups 15, 19, 29
medically unexplained
    symptoms 16
meditation 81, 85
melatonin 13, 91, 135, 136
memory loss 44, 45
menopause 38, 39, 129
methotrexate 35
methylcellulose 27
mind-body medicine 99
minerals 35, 58–63, 93, 94
movements 30
MSM (methyl sulphonyl
    methane) 59, 60
muscles 66, 82, 83
myocardial infarction 24

N

nail care 95
native American Indian herbs
    124
naturopathy 29, 35, 39, 45,
    130–132

nicotine replacement therapy
    (NRT) 21
nonsteroidal anti-inflammatory
    drugs 34
noradrenaline 78
nutrition 27, 54–57
nutritional therapy 35, 37, 39,
    57

O

obesity 27, 28
optimum heart rate 65, 66
Oriental massage 104, 105
orlistat 27
osteoarthritis 34
osteopathy 31, 108–111
osteoporosis 36, 37

P

painkillers 31
Palmer, Daniel David 108
paracetamol 31, 34
Patanjali 114
pelvic floor exercises 43
penicillamine 35
phentermine 27
physiotherapy 31
plastic surgery 138, 139
posture 30, 32, 74–77, 108,
    111
prazosin 41
presbycusis 49
presbyopia 48, 49
preventive measures 15
processed food 55
progesterone 13, 38
prostate problems 40, 41
protein 55
psychotherapy 21, 39, 81

R

raloxifene 37
reflexology 81, 112, 113
relaxation 39, 43, 81–87
rheumatoid arthritis 34
rivastigmine 45
Rolfing 76, 77

S

salt 22, 24, 55, 62
salute the sun 118, 119
saturated fats 23
sedatives 20
selective alpha-blockers 41
sex therapy 42
sibutramine 27
sight problems 46, 47
sildenafil 42
sitting twist 33

skin care 92–95
sleep 45, 80, 88–91
smoking 20, 21, 22, 80
snoring 90
social isolation 52, 80
soy supplements 39
spiritual practices 80
sport 72, 73
sports massage 104, 105
standing twist 33
Still, Andrew Taylor 108
stress 22, 24, 65, 78–81
sugar 54, 55
sulfonylurea 29
supplements 58–63
support groups 80
surgery 35, 41
synthetic catalytic scavengers
    136, 137

T

Tai chi 37, 45, 81
telomerase 13
telomerase-based drugs 137
testosterone 13, 136
thiamine 59, 60
time management 80, 81
tinnitus 49
tissue salts 129

V

valium 81
varicose veins 25
vegetables 54, 56, 57
visualization 81, 86
vitamins 36, 37, 58–63,
    93–94

W

walking 66, 72
water 56
weight 15, 22, 24, 27, 53,
    57
weight training 73
well-being 65
Western herbalism 123
wrinkles 92, 93

Y

yoga 25, 29, 32, 37, 45,
    81, 114–119

Z

zinc 40, 41, 59, 63